Operative Surgery

MANUAL

Vijay P. Khatri, MD, FACS

Assistant Professor of Surgery
Department of Surgery
Division of Surgical Oncology
University of California, Davis, Medical Center
Sacramento, California

Juan A. Asensio, MD, FACS

Unit Chief, Trauma Surgery Service A
Division of Trauma Surgery and
 Surgical Critical Care
Department of Surgery
Associate Professor and Senior Attending Surgeon
University of Southern California
 Keck School of Medicine
Senior Attending Surgeon
The Los Angeles County/University of
 Southern California Medical Center
Los Angeles, California

SAUNDERS
An Imprint of Elsevier Science (USA)
Philadelphia London New York St. Louis Sydney Toronto

SAUNDERS
An Imprint of Elsevier Science (USA)

The Curtis Center
Independence Square West
Philadelphia, Pennsylvania 19106

OPERATIVE SURGERY MANUAL ISBN 0–7216–7864–5

NOTICE

Library of Congress Cataloging-in-Publication Data
Khatri, Vijay P.
    Operative surgery manual / Vijay P. Khatri, Juan A. Asensio.
    p.; cm.
    ISBN 0–7216–7864–5
    1. Surgery, Operative–Handbooks, manuals, etc. I. Asensio, Juan A. II. Title.
    [DNLM: 1. Surgical Procedures, Operative–Handbooks. WO 39 K45o 2003]
    RD32 .K45 2003
    617'.91–dc21 2002075768

Acquisitions Editor: Joe Rusko
Project Manager: Amy Norwitz
Cover/Book Designer: Ellen Zanolle
CE/MVY

Printed in the United States of America
Last digit is the print number: 9 8 7 6 5 4 3 2 1

To my parents, my wife Anjana, and children Amit and Shevani, and to the memory of my grandfather, Govindbhai Khatri
VPK

To my family—Elsa, Juan Carlos, Alex Ariel, and Strella—and to the memory of my parents, Olga and Jose Alfredo Asensio
JAA

Foreword

Hamlet confides to Rosencrantz and Guildenstern, *"What a piece of work is a man, how noble in reason, how infinite in faculties, in form and moving how express and admirable, in action how like an angel."* It is the treasured province and privilege of surgeons to visit in the flesh that express and admirable form. With reverence, humility, and intent to do good, the visitation is an act of grace. With knowledge and skill, there is joy in the exercise. With the anatomy intimately familiar, such journeys are a visit to old friends. When beginning a career of these journeys, nothing is more essential than a first-class guide. Drs. Khatri and Asensio and Elsevier Science have obliged in the publication of this succinct and well-constructed manual. It is a companion, designed to be where the young surgeon finds himself or herself, there where it is needed. The convenience of this manual should not belie the wealth of information it contains. It is a rich source, articulate and approachable in what it has to tell. It is designed to be read or to be consulted frequently for review.

The presentation of each operative procedure begins with a lucid exposition of the pertinent anatomy, the indispensable cornerstone of the surgeon's practical knowledge. Adding the embryology is more than a subtle nicety. It is a reminder of critical three-dimensional relationships. Informative pearls to make the patient ready for surgery are there for the taking. Emphasis is given to operative procedure, so essential to a successful working environment for a surgical procedure. Operations performed well are those in which the surgeon can comfortably see and work. Creating this opportunity is a matter of knowledge and experience. The procedure descriptions reflect a broad experience at the operating table translated into fluent, clear English, a good read for the novice and experienced alike. The illustrations complement the text.

This manual covers the core of general surgery and provides the student of surgery (at any career level) advice on most procedures performed by general surgeons. Information provided can be extended to procedures not included. The text is a window to the extensive experience of Dr. Khatri, who has trained in and taught surgery on both sides of the Atlantic. He has an abiding interest in the craft of surgery and in teaching it, and no less skill in rendering his thoughts and ideas into print. This manual is a guide on which the student or surgeon in training can build personal experience and more readily absorb the advice and teaching of his or her mentor. It is also a guide for the experienced who are diligently preparing themselves to revisit some part of the express and admirable form. It will be a valued companion on the journey.

James E. Goodnight, MD, PhD
Pearl Stamps Stewart Chair
Professor and Chairman, Department of Surgery
University of California, Davis, Medical Center
Sacramento, California

Foreword

As you are reading this foreword, you may be thinking that we do not need another manual demonstrating surgical techniques. However, Khatri and Asensio, the authors of this particular operative surgery manual, have created something that did not exist before. For surgical residents or medical students embarking on a surgical rotation or a general surgery residency program, this operative surgery manual is invaluable.

Khatri and Asensio have done a fine job in covering the major anatomic sites, which are described in a way that provides a quick knowledge base and a feel for the specific surgical procedure. It is difficult to use a large operative textbook as a reference to prepare for the next day's surgical procedures if one is preparing for three or four cases. *Operative Surgery Manual* is a practical book, which succinctly describes the operative technique in a simple narrative form with key illustrations. The manual is small enough that it can be carried in the pocket of the resident or medical student to be readily available on call to prepare for any emergency case.

Because in all training programs in the United States there is a long gap between the time anatomy is taught in the first year of medical school and the resident's surgical rotations, Khatri and Asensio have added clinically relevant anatomy and embryology in each of the sections described. Therefore, the residents and medical students can have easy access under one cover to information on anatomy, embryology, and operative technique. A focused preoperative preparation section is also included.

Vijay P. Khatri, MD, is well qualified to have put this operative surgery manual together. Aside from his general surgery training, he has been a National Institutes of Health T32 Laboratory Research Fellow at the Roswell Park Cancer Institute in Buffalo, New York, and has had additional training in surgical oncology at the same institution. His experience as a teacher and mentor to medical students and surgical residents is evident in this manual.

Nicholas J. Petrelli, MD
MBNA Endowed Medical Director
Helen F. Graham Cancer Center
Newark, Delaware
Professor of Surgery
Thomas Jefferson Medical College
Philadelphia, Pennsylvania

Preface

Surgery does the ideal thing—it separates the patient from his disease. It puts the patient back to bed and the disease in a bottle.

Logan Clendening (1884–1945)

The fundamental goal in the creation of the *Operative Surgery Manual* was to provide surgical trainees and medical students with a practical guide to commonly encountered surgical procedures. Much emphasis has been placed on maintaining a standardized format throughout the manual to allow the reader to predict the flow of the chapters. The detailed narrative text is complemented with illustrations created by a single artist to maintain a uniform presentation style and conceptual consistency that facilitates comprehension of the operative procedure.

The major purpose of the *Operative Surgery Manual* is to bring to the reader a "one-stop" reference including embryology, anatomic facts of practical value, focused preoperative preparation, and a concise description of contemporary operative technique. Furthermore, as a reasonably sized book it can be carried in the pocket and be readily available to review surgical technique before scrubbing for the operation.

To prepare for operative procedures, often surgical residents have needed to refer to surgical texts that contain encyclopedic amounts of surgical knowledge that can be difficult to cover expeditiously. Alternatively, a surgical atlas that has exhaustive illustrations accompanied by brief text cannot convey the subtleties of operative technique. In the *Operative Surgery Manual*, we present a succinct yet detailed narrative of surgical techniques, which we hope can familiarize the reader with the essential elements of the operative procedures. Furthermore, we recognized that for most surgical residents and medical students, several years have passed since their anatomy lectures during the first year of medical school. Knowledge of surgical anatomy represents a critical foundation for students embarking on a surgical rotation and even more so for surgical trainees. The importance of anatomy was well expressed by one of my surgical teachers, who stated, "If you know what structures to save, the rest can go." This lighthearted but poignant statement has remained an important aphorism for one of the authors' (VPK) successful approach to complex multiorgan resections in surgical oncology.

Being knowledgeable of the essential facts of human development greatly clarifies gross anatomy. However, to refresh his or her knowledge of anatomy and embryology, the reader may need to refer to yet another textbook.

The *Operative Surgery Manual* has been organized into 7 major sections with 50 chapters. The large section on Abdomen has been further divided into anatomic site subsections: *abdominal wall, esophagus/ stomach/duodenum/small bowel, hepatobiliary system, pancreas, spleen,* and *large bowel/anorectum*. Each chapter contains relevant embryology, surgical anatomy, and the operative procedure. The surgical procedure is divided according to the important phases for expeditious conduct of the operation: *position, incision, exposure and operative technique,* and *closure*. This format has been maintained throughout the textbook to provide consistency to the reader. Several chapters discussing emergency operations have been included: *perforated peptic ulcer, bleeding duodenal ulcer, esophageal perforation, appendectomy,* and *femoral embolectomy*. Advanced operative procedures such as *radical and modified radical neck dissection, Ivor-Lewis esophagectomy, radical gastrectomy, pancreatico-duodenectomy (Whipple procedure), hepatic resection, subtotal colectomy/ panproctocolectomy and J-pouch reconstruction,* and *radical cystectomy* are just some of the chapters that senior trainees should find particularly informative.

To maintain our objective of keeping this textbook a handy manual, we have selected routine operations that will be encountered on a day-to-day basis by the surgical trainee. Although there has been an explosion in advanced laparoscopic surgery, we have limited our coverage to the most commonly performed laparoscopic procedures. We welcome comments from readers regarding topics they believe would further enhance the *Manual's* utility.

This book reflects our passion as surgical educators and our hope that it finds itself a unique niche as a learning resource for medical students and surgical trainees at all levels.

Vijay P. Khatri, MD, FACS

Juan A. Asensio, MD, FACS

Acknowledgments

Although the *Operative Surgery Manual* represents an individualistic approach to surgical technique, we acknowledge that this work could not have been completed without enormous contributions by various individuals. We are grateful for the energetic editing by Shirley Cable, whose enthusiasm and attention to every sentence has enhanced the *Manual's* clarity. The text has been admirably complemented with high-quality illustrations by Peggy Firth.

We extend our appreciation to Lisette Bralow, Elsevier Science, for supporting our vision and shepherding us through the conceptual plans and subsequent development of the textbook. Joe Rusko, Acquisitions Editor at Elsevier Science, has been instrumental during the ever important last sprint towards successful completion of the *Operative Surgery Manual*. Appreciation is due also to Amy Norwitz and the production staff at Elsevier Science for their tireless efforts during the final assembly. Thanks also go to Sandra Moura, Jackie Stout, and Espie Gutierrez, who have been responsible for much of the correspondence during the final phase of the textbook and needless to say for the preservation of our sanity. We also owe a great deal to our patients for their trust and acknowledge the residents and medical students for their intellectual stimulation and curiosity that inspire us to be better educators.

Finally, we would like to thank our spouses, who have been extremely supportive during the entire preparation of this text.

Contents

Vascular Surgery

Urology

Gynecology

Head and Neck Surgery

CHAPTER 1

Thyroidectomy

EMBRYOLOGY During the fourth week of fetal development, an endodermal thickening develops in the floor of the primitive pharynx at the junctional area between the first and second pharyngeal pouches called the foramen cecum. The endodermal thickening, which represents the primitive thyroid tissue, penetrates the underlying mesenchymal tissue and begins to descend anterior to the hyoid bone and the laryngeal cartilages to reach its final adult position in front of the trachea. The thyroid diverticulum becomes bilobed and develops into two lateral lobes and a median isthmus. The thyroid gland is temporarily attached to the lumen of the foregut at the foramen cecum by the thyroglossal duct, which eventually solidifies and disappears. The distal portion of the thyroglossal duct gives rise to the pyramidal lobe and the levator superioris thyroideae in adults. Ectopic thyroid tissue can be found at any point along its embryologic descent.

ANATOMY The thyroid gland weighs about 25 g and is composed of two lobes attached by the isthmus. The isthmus is related posteriorly to the second, third, and fourth tracheal rings; knowledge of this relation is pertinent during the performance of tracheostomy. A variable-sized pyramidal lobe arises from the isthmus and is directed upward usually to the left, although it may be absent in 50% of individuals. The gland lies on the anterolateral aspect of the cervical trachea and extends from the level of the thyroid cartilage to the fifth or sixth tracheal ring. Anteriorly it is covered by the pretracheal fascia, strap muscles, and, more laterally, the sternocleidomastoid muscle. The blood supply to the thyroid gland is derived from (1) the superior thyroid artery, which arises from the external carotid artery and descends to the upper pole of the gland; (2) the inferior thyroid artery, a branch of the thyrocervical trunk that arises from the subclavian artery; and (3) the inconsistently present thyroidea ima artery, arising from the innominate artery, right subclavian artery, or aortic arch. Venous drainage is from the (1) superior thyroid vein, which drains directly into the internal jugular vein, (2) middle thyroid vein, which drains into the internal jugular vein and is the first vessel encountered during thyroidectomy, and (3) inferior thyroid vein, which leaves the lower border of the gland to join the left innominate vein (Fig. 1–1).

Several important structures are in close relation to the gland and are of surgical relevance. The external laryngeal nerve, a branch of the superior laryngeal nerve, accompanies the superior thyroid pedicle and travels medially to supply the cricothyroid muscle. If this nerve is severed, it alters the voice pitch, which is particularly important to singers. The recurrent laryngeal nerve is a branch of the vagus, and embryologically it arises in close relation to the fourth aortic arch. Because of the descent of the fourth aortic arch vessels (the subclavian artery on the right and the aortic arch on the left), the recurrent nerves first are drawn caudally into the mediastinum and then course upward toward their final destination, the vocal cords. The nerve usually lies in the tracheoesophageal groove near the terminal branches of the inferior thyroid artery (see Fig. 1–1). The recurrent laryngeal nerve is usually found in Simon's triangle, which is formed by the inferior thyroid artery superiorly, the common carotid artery laterally, and the esophagus medially. The surgeon also needs to be aware of the presence of a nonrecurrent laryngeal nerve. The posterior aspect of each thyroid lobe is related to the parathyroid glands and is at risk of injury during thyroidectomy. The anatomy of the parathyroid glands is described in Chapter 2.

SPECIAL PREPARATION Apart from ordering routine investigations and reviewing special investigations that may have been performed, such as thyroid function tests, ultrasonography of the thyroid, isotope scan, and fine-needle aspiration, cytology must be reviewed. Serum calcium level is obtained because hyperparathyroidism may coexist.

Indirect laryngoscopy is performed preoperatively to evaluate the mobility of the vocal cords and detect unsuspected vocal cord paralysis (if paralysis is present, it is essential not to damage the recurrent laryngeal nerve supplying the normal vocal cords). Patients who are thyrotoxic should be rendered euthyroid. This can be achieved medically by the use of carbimazole. If the patient has evidence of sympathetic overdrive such as tachycardia, a beta-blocker such as propranolol is added but must be continued postoperatively for 8 to 10 days. There is no need to use iodides,

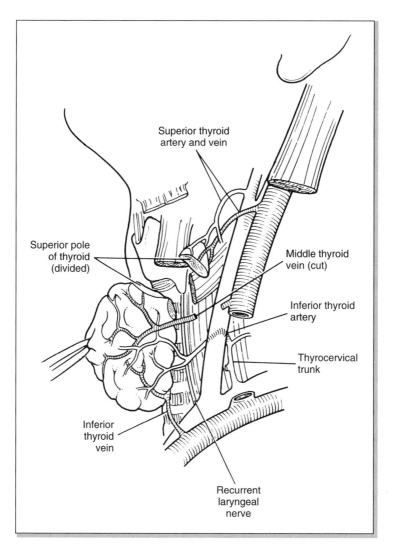

FIGURE 1–1 Blood supply of the thyroid gland and the important adjacent anatomic structures.

because there is no convincing evidence that it reduces vascularity of the thyroid gland.

Operative Procedure

POSITION The patient is placed in a supine position initially with the neck extended by placing a ring beneath the head and a sandbag roll beneath the shoulder. The patient is placed in a reverse Trendelenburg position. The neck and the upper thorax are prepped, and a head towel is placed. To maintain sterility on the lateral aspect of the neck, folded towels are placed. Next, four towels are placed and secured to the skin with either silk sutures or towel clips. The surgeon stands on the side opposite to the lobe that is being resected.

INCISION The incision is marked 2 to 3 cm above the sternal notch along a skin crease using an indelible pen. A very low incision can lead to a keloid scar and fixes the skin onto bony prominences. The lateral ends of the incision are curved to follow Langer lines and must be symmetrical. The incision should extend the same distance on each side of midline and usually continues beyond the anterior border of the sternocleidomastoid muscle. Shorter incisions not only provide inadequate exposure but may contract and thus be cosmetically unappealing. To avoid excessive dermal bleeding, the incision can be infiltrated with 1% lidocaine containing epinephrine. With a no. 15 scalpel the skin and subcutaneous tissues are sharply divided and the platysma identified. The platysma is then divided with electrocautery.

EXPOSURE AND OPERATIVE TECHNIQUE Once the platysma is divided, the assistant lifts the skin and the platysma upward with double skin hooks to allow for the creation of a subplatysmal flap. Maintaining the dissection close to the platysma ensures that cervical fascia is not included in the flap. The superior flap extends upward to the thyroid notch and the lower flap extends downward to the sternal notch. This procedure should be blood free, because the superficial veins lie beneath the cervical fascia. To retract the skin flaps, either Weitlaner or Gelpi retractors can be used.

After the flaps are created, the key to this operation is locating the correct plane of dissection. Next, the investing fascia is opened in the midline between the anterior jugular veins; this opening extends from the thyroid cartilage superiorly to the suprasternal notch inferiorly. At the lower part there is usually a transverse cervical vein that needs to be clamped, divided, and ligated with 3-0 silk sutures. The strap muscles (the sternohyoid, and deep to that, the sternothyroid) are carefully dissected to allow their retraction laterally. At times these muscles may need to be transected to gain better access to the thyroid gland; when necessary this should be done at the level of the thyroid cartilage to preserve their innervation from the ansa hypoglossi nerve (Fig. 1–2). If there is local invasion by a thyroid neoplasm, the thyroid lobe is resected en bloc with its overlying strap muscles.

Dissecting close to the strap muscles minimizes bleeding. The correct plane of dissection is entered when the vessels overlying the thyroid gland become prominent. The loose areolar tissue overlying the thyroid gland is

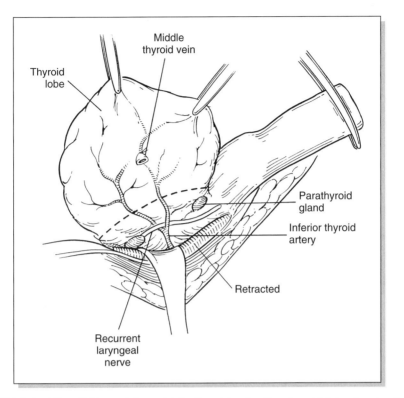

FIGURE 1–2 After division of the middle thyroid vein, the thyroid lobe is retracted medially to expose the parathyroid glands, recurrent laryngeal nerve, and inferior thyroid artery.

divided with electrocautery. Blunt dissection on the lateral aspect of the thyroid gland must be avoided, as it invariably leads to bleeding because here the vessels are friable and tear easily. After the anterior surface of the thyroid has been thoroughly exposed, the entire gland is carefully explored and palpated.

The strap muscles are firmly retracted with a small loop retractor while the thyroid gland is drawn medially. To permit further medial rotation of the thyroid gland, the next step involves division of the middle thyroid vein after ligating it in continuity with 3-0 silk sutures (see Fig. 1–2). The silk tie on the distal aspect of the vein can be left long to aid in further subcapsular dissection. The capsule along the lateral border of the thyroid gland is dissected with fine Halsted mosquito hemostats and divided with bipolar electrocautery. Further mobilization of the thyroid gland to improve exposure of the posterior surface can only be obtained by dissecting the superior pole. With a retractor, the upper portion of the strap muscles is drawn cephalad. Concurrently, the thyroid gland is firmly retracted downward.

With use of a Kittner dissector and a Jackson right-angle clamp, the upper pole is separated from the cricothyroid muscle, to which the external branch of the superior laryngeal nerve is adherent. The lateral portion of the upper pole is also freed. The terminal branches of the superior thyroid artery and vein are identified, ligated in continuity with 2-0 silk sutures, and divided. If necessary, two ligatures are placed proximally, because once divided the superior thyroid artery tends to retract. Do not mass-ligate the superior pole, because it will endanger the external laryngeal nerve.

After division of the superior thyroid pole, the thyroid gland can be easily rotated medially. Attention is now directed toward identifying the parathyroid glands and the recurrent laryngeal nerve (see Fig. 1–2). Parathyroid glands are small, yellowish brown, and soft and pliable, in contrast to lymph nodes or thyroid nodules, which are firm. Furthermore, a single small artery can be seen entering the gland; the artery radiates out over the capsule in a fernlike pattern. The upper parathyroid gland is invariably found behind the upper third of the thyroid gland adjacent to the cricothyroid junction.

Next, the carotid artery is identified and retracted laterally. At approximately the junction of the middle and lower thirds of the thyroid gland, the tortuous inferior thyroid artery is identified, which helps locate the recurrent laryngeal nerve. Often a triangle (Simon's triangle) is formed by the common carotid artery laterally, inferior thyroid artery superiorly, and esophagus medially, and the recurrent laryngeal nerve can be seen coursing upward in this triangle to enter the larynx. The nerve usually appears as a white cord with fine red vasa vasorum coursing over its surface. Dissection should proceed directly over the recurrent laryngeal nerve to expose it along its course to the larynx. If the recurrent laryngeal nerve remains difficult to identify, the possibility of a nonrecurrent laryngeal nerve should be considered.

The inferior parathyroid gland should be identified next; it is usually found adjacent to the terminal branch of the inferior thyroid artery on the posterior surface of the thyroid. Once the integrity of the recurrent laryngeal nerve and the parathyroid glands has been ensured, the terminal branches of the inferior thyroid artery close to the thyroid capsule are ligated. Ligation of the main trunk of the inferior thyroid artery should be avoided, because it compromises the blood supply of the parathyroid glands.

Dissection now proceeds around the lower pole of the thyroid. The pole is mobilized by careful dissection with a combination of Kittner dissector, Halsted mosquitoes, or Jackson right-angle clamp, and all blood vessels entering are divided and ligated using 3-0 silk sutures. These maneuvers facilitate further medial rotation of the thyroid gland. For total lobectomy, the thyroid lobe and the isthmus are dissected off the anterolateral wall of the trachea while the recurrent laryngeal nerve is kept under direct vision. A straight Crile clamp is placed between the isthmus and the opposite lobe, and the specimen is sharply excised. The thyroid tissue within the clamp is oversewn with a running interlocking 3-0 silk suture for hemostasis.

If a total thyroidectomy is being performed, the remaining lobe is removed in a similar fashion, with division of the middle thyroid vein, identification of the recurrent laryngeal nerve and parathyroid glands, and ligation and division of the superior pole and branches of the inferior thyroid vessels.

CLOSURE The operative area is irrigated, and hemostasis is achieved. To control troublesome oozing, instead of using electrocautery, topical hemostatic agents such as Gelfoam, thrombin, or Surgicel are used because they do not endanger adjacent vital structures. A Valsalva maneuver is performed on the patient by the anesthesiologist, and the operative area is again carefully checked for hemostasis; if achieved, there is no need for a drain.

To help with wound closure, the neck is brought into neutral position by removal of the shoulder roll. The deep cervical fascia in the midline is sutured with 3-0 absorbable sutures. For a good cosmetic result, the platysma must be carefully reapproximated with interrupted 3-0 absorbable sutures. The skin can be closed with subcuticular 4-0 nonabsorbable monofilament or absorbable sutures.

CHAPTER 2

Parathyroidectomy

EMBRYOLOGY The inferior parathyroid glands develop from the dorsal bud of the third pharyngeal pouch, whereas the superior parathyroid glands are derived from the fourth pharyngeal pouch. These glands attach to the dorsal surface of the thyroid gland as it migrates caudally. Parathyroid glands derived from the third pharyngeal pouch come to lie in a more inferior position because they descend along with the thymus gland (which is derived from the ventral bud of the third pharyngeal pouch). Failure of the formation of the parathyroid gland and thymus from the third pharyngeal pouch results in the DiGeorge syndrome. Variations in embryologic migration can result in ectopic parathyroid tissue. Knowledge of these sites is essential during the performance of parathyroidectomy.

ANATOMY The number of parathyroid glands may vary from two to six, but in 90% of patients there are four (two on each side). Each gland is oval, approximately 6 mm long, and frequently covered with adipose tissue. These glands are related to the posterior surface of the thyroid gland and often lie within its fascial covering. The two superior parathyroid glands are more constant in location and can be found at about the level of the cricoid cartilage. The two inferior parathyroid glands are more variable in location, although they frequently lie along the lower part of the thyroid gland. The blood supply to these glands is from an upper and a lower parathyroid artery that arise from the inferior thyroid artery. On rare occasions, the upper parathyroid artery can arise from the superior thyroid artery.

SPECIAL PREOPERATIVE PREPARATION   Before exploration, the basic labora-tory tests that should be reviewed are the total ionized serum calcium, phosphate, alkaline phosphatase, and protein levels. Elevated levels of parathyroid hormone should be confirmed. Preoperative localization studies are not required, although high-resolution ultrasonography or nuclear medicine scintigraphy, including thallium/technetium subtraction scan and sestamibi scan, may be obtained and may be helpful. Preoperative laryngoscopy is performed routinely to rule out occult vocal cord paralysis.

Operative Procedure

POSITION   The patient is usually placed in a supine position, and the neck is extended either by placing the head on a ring or by placing a rolled towel beneath the shoulders. The neck and the upper thorax are scrubbed, prepped, and draped in the usual manner. The patient is placed in reverse Trendelenburg position.

INCISION   A curvilinear transverse skin-crease incision is marked with an indelible pen approximately two fingers-breadth above the clavicle. The skin at the proposed site of incision is infiltrated with 1% lidocaine with epinephrine. The skin incision is made and deepened with electrocautery until the platysma is identified.

EXPOSURE AND OPERATIVE TECHNIQUE   The platysma is divided with electro-cautery, and subplatysmal flaps are developed superiorly and inferiorly. The midline is identified and the cervical fascia incised. The strap muscles are dissected off the thyroid gland and retracted laterally. Beginning on either the right or the left side or the side indicated by preoperative imag-ing, the thyroid lobe is elevated and rotated medially. The areolar tissue is carefully cleared from around the lobe, and the inferior thyroid artery and the recurrent laryngeal nerves are identified. It is important to expose the nerve from its entrance into the operative field to the level of the larynx. As a rule, it is safer to expose vital structures so that they are identified and preserved rather than avoiding their exposure and iatrogenically damaging them. It is essential to avoid unnecessary bleeding in the operative field because it can make the identification of parathyroid glands difficult. The parathyroid glands characteristically are yellowish brown and vary in shape and dimension. The thyroid tissue is usually red, lymph nodes are paler and pinker, and thymic tissue is pale grayish yellow. The parathyroid gland is also identified by observing a single small artery entering its hilus and radiating out over the capsule. The usual number of parathyroid glands is four, although five parathyroid glands can be found in 4% of cases, three in 5% of cases, and two in less than 1%. The anatomic location of the parathyroid glands is reasonably constant (Fig. 2–1). In approximately 80% of the cases, the glands are situated symmetrically on opposite sides of the neck. The superior parathyroid glands are invariably found behind the upper pole of the thyroid gland or at the cricothyroid junction. The inferior parathyroid glands can be variable in location due to embryologic mobility but are generally found in the immediate vicinity of the lower pole of the thyroid. The surgeon should identify all parathyroid glands before removing any of them, however; some surgeons perform preoperative localization and explore and resect only the enlarged parathyroid gland(s).

If an inferior parathyroid gland cannot be found after an extensive search in the operative area, the thymus should be gently elevated from the mediastinum. If the parathyroid gland still cannot be located, in addition

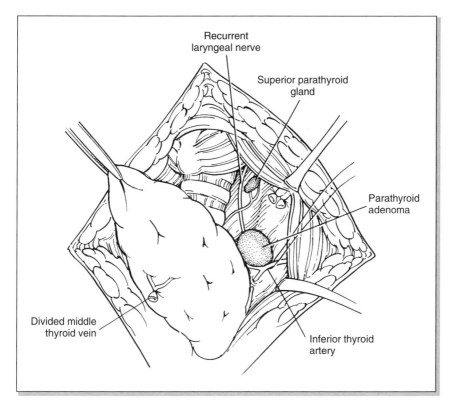

FIGURE 2–1 Location of the inferior parathyroid adenoma adjacent to the inferior thyroid artery and recurrent laryngeal nerve. The superior parathyroid gland is invariably found behind the upper pole of the thyroid gland or at the cricothyroid junction.

to examining the thyrothymic ligament, the surgeon should examine the tracheoesophageal groove, retroesophageal space, and carotid sheath to locate an ectopic parathyroid gland. The key anatomic structures are the inferior thyroid artery and its branches, which will often guide the surgeon to the parathyroid glands (see Fig. 2–1). If three parathyroid glands have been identified and one is enlarged and the other two are of normal size, an extensive search is undertaken. If the fourth gland cannot be found, the procedure may be terminated because the chance of leaving behind a second hyperfunctioning parathyroid gland is approximately 5% to 10%. If, on the other hand, two or more enlarged parathyroid glands have been identified and the fourth gland cannot be found, a diligent search is necessary because the likelihood that the remaining fourth gland is enlarged is greater than 50%.

If the retroesophageal and retropharyngeal spaces and the carotid sheath have been explored and the fourth gland still has not been identified, an ipsilateral thyroid lobectomy should be considered if the diagnosis of parathyroid hyperplasia is considered. At the initial exploration, one should not proceed with a sternotomy but should terminate the cervical exploration and then proceed to confirm the diagnosis by performing localizing studies before undertaking a mediastinal dissection. Once the surgeon has identified the parathyroid glands, the extent of resection is based on the operative findings. When an adenoma is found and normal glands are identified, only the adenoma needs to be removed to cure hyperparathyroidism. Biopsy of all three remaining glands is unnecessary and undesirable because it can lead to ischemic injury.

If four hyperplastic glands are identified, the surgeon has the option of performing a subtotal parathyroidectomy, in which approximately 35 to 50 mg of one parathyroid gland is left in situ. Alternatively, a total parathyroidectomy with immediate transplantation of the parathyroid tissue in either the sternocleidomastoid or the forearm muscles may be performed. The remaining parathyroid gland, whether in the neck or in the forearm, should be marked with hemoclips for subsequent identification if hyperparathyroidism recurs. If four normal parathyroid glands are found, the surgeon has to diligently search for an adenoma of a supernumerary gland elsewhere in the neck, as described earlier, or within the thyrothymic ligament or thymus itself.

If at the time of surgery the enlarged parathyroid gland feels hard and appears grayish in color and is firmly fixed to surrounding tissue, the possibility of parathyroid carcinoma should be entertained. In this situation it is often necessary to perform an ipsilateral thyroid lobectomy and resection of the parathyroid tumor and the adjacent invading structures. If there are enlarged lymph nodes, a neck dissection may also be needed.

CLOSURE The wound is irrigated and hemostasis is secured. Routine drainage is usually unnecessary. The platysma is carefully reapproximated with interrupted 3-0 absorbable sutures. The dermis is closed with interrupted 3-0 absorbable sutures and the skin is approximated with 4-0 subcuticular nonabsorbable monofilament or absorbable sutures. Steri-Strips are applied longitudinally, which can act as a dressing as well.

CHAPTER 3

Tracheostomy

EMBRYOLOGY See Chapter 7 for a full description of the development of the lungs.

ANATOMY The trachea is about 10 cm long and 2 cm in diameter and extends from the larynx at the level of the sixth cervical vertebra to its bifurcation into two bronchi at the level of the fourth thoracic vertebra. It is composed of numerous incomplete cartilaginous rings that are united posteriorly with membranous tissue to form the membranous portion of the trachea.

Anteriorly, the pretracheal fascia, the isthmus of the thyroid gland, and the infrahyoid strap muscles cover the trachea. The esophagus lies posterior to the trachea, with the recurrent laryngeal nerve situated in the tracheoesophageal groove. The common carotid artery laterally, inferior thyroid artery superiorly, and esophagus medially form Simons triangle. The lateral relations of the trachea are the lateral lobes of the thyroid gland, the inferior thyroid artery, and the carotid sheath with its contents.

The blood supply of the trachea is from the inferior thyroid vessels, and its lymphatic drainage is to paratracheal lymph nodes.

Operative Technique

POSITION The patient is placed in the supine position, and the neck is extended with a shoulder roll. General anesthesia is administered with endotracheal intubation. The neck and upper thorax are prepped and draped in the usual fashion.

INCISION　Approximately two fingers-breadth above the suprasternal notch, a 4- to 6-cm transverse incision is marked (Fig. 3–1*A*).

EXPOSURE AND OPERATIVE TECHNIQUE　An incision is sharply made and carried through the subcutaneous tissue and the platysma. Self-retaining Weitlaner retractors are placed longitudinally and transversely. The midline cervical fascia is identified and divided longitudinally. The anterior jugular veins are avoided if possible; if necessary they are ligated in continuity with 3-0 silk sutures and divided. Next, the underlying sternothyroid is also retracted laterally with two Army-Navy retractors. Dissection should be kept in the midline heading directly toward the trachea. If the thyroid isthmus lies over the second or third tracheal ring, it can be either retracted upward or divided. Division of the isthmus is often needed, where the thyroid tissue is dissected with a Mixter right-angle clamp, divided, and transfixed with 2-0 silk suture ligatures. To maintain exposure, the two Weitlaner retractors are repositioned as the dissection proceeds toward the trachea.

The thyroid cartilage notch and more inferiorly the cricothyroid membrane and the cricoid cartilage are identified. The second and third tracheal rings are identified and marked lightly with electrocautery. Before opening the trachea, ensure that a suction catheter is available. Also ensure that the tracheostomy cuff is intact and well lubricated. A cruciate incision is made sharply between the second and third tracheal rings, and the edges are separated with a tracheal retractor (Fig. 3–1*B*). Placing the tracheostomy more inferiorly can increase the risk of pressure on the innominate artery and thus the risk of tracheoinnominate fistula. The surgeon must also be aware of the presence of the thyroid ima artery (in 13% of patients) arising from the aortic arch and of the thyroid ima vein (in 13% of patients) draining into the innominate vein to avoid iatrogenic injury to these vessels.

After placement of the tracheostomy, the anesthesiologist is requested to withdraw the endotracheal tube, and the tracheostomy tube is gently slipped into the trachea. The end of the tracheal tube is completely withdrawn, and the ventilator is connected to the tracheostomy after the blunt obturator is removed. Mucus should be suctioned from the tracheobronchial tree.

CLOSURE　Secure the flange of the tracheostomy to the skin with four corner sutures using 3-0 monofilament sutures. Because the skin incision is usually small, only one or two interrupted 4-0 monofilament sutures are required to approximate the skin. To further secure the tracheostomy, a narrow umbilical tape is placed loosely around the patient's neck and attached to the tracheostomy flange. A gauze dressing is placed at the side of the tracheostomy.

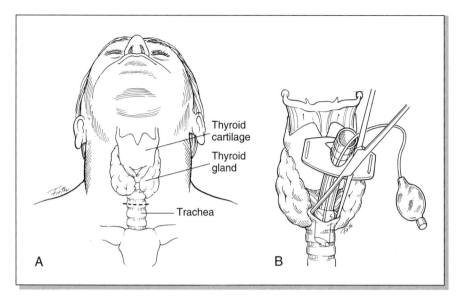

Thyroid
cartilage

Thyroid
gland

Trachea

A

B

FIGURE 3–1 *A*, The transverse incision is shown in relation to the underlying bony structures. *B*, After the thyroid isthmus is retracted superiorly, the tracheostomy tube is inserted with the assistance of the tracheal retractor.

CHAPTER 4

Parotidectomy

EMBRYOLOGY   The epithelial lining of the primitive mouth gives rise to solid buds that develop into the parotid glands. The surrounding capsule is derived from the adjacent mesenchymal tissue. The basal motor plate of the myelencephalon contains the dorsal nucleus of the vagus and the inferior salivatory nucleus, which innervate the parotid gland via the glossopharyngeal nerve.

ANATOMY   The parotid gland is the largest of the paired salivary glands. It is a wedge-shaped gland located in a compact area that is bounded by the following bony structures: the ramus of the mandible anteriorly, the mastoid process posteriorly, and the styloid process medially. Skin and the deep investing cervical fascia cover the superficial surface of the gland. The posteromedial surface of the gland lies on the mastoid process, the sternocleidomastoid, and the posterior belly of digastric muscle. The anteromedial surface extends over the masseter muscle laterally and the medial pterygoid muscle medially. The deep surface of the gland is intimately related to the styloid process and its attached muscles. Emerging from the anterior border of the parotid gland is the parotid duct (Stenson's duct), which passes over the masseter muscle and then dives immediately to pierce the buccal mucosa and opens opposite the upper second molar tooth. The structures that lie within the parotid gland from the medial to the lateral aspect are (1) the external carotid artery, (2) the retromandibular vein, (3) the facial nerve, and (4) the lymph nodes lying immediately beneath the parotid fascia. The facial nerve, which is the nerve of the second pharyngeal arch, emerges from the stylomastoid foramen and enters the parotid gland, where it divides into five branches that supply the muscles of facial expression. These five branches are the temporal, zygomatic, buccal, marginal mandibular, and cervical.

The arterial supply of the parotid gland is derived from the external carotid artery. The venous drainage flows into the retromandibular vein. The sympathetic supply to the parotid gland is from the superior cervical ganglion. The parasympathetic fibers from the inferior salivary nucleus of the glossopharyngeal nerve reach the parotid gland via the otic ganglion and auriculotemporal nerve.

PREOPERATIVE PREPARATION   Apart from basic investigations, the imaging studies of the parotid gland, particularly the computed tomography scan, must be reviewed, although parotidectomy is usually based on clinical suspicion and the results of fine-needle aspiration cytology. Preoperatively the function of the facial nerve must be confirmed to be intact by physical examination. Informed consent, informing the patient about the risks of damage to the facial nerve, loss of sensation over the earlobe, and the potential for gustatory sweating over the parotidectomy area, must be obtained.

Operative Procedure

POSITION   The patient undergoes general anesthesia with endotracheal intubation, but anesthesiologists must refrain from using paralyzing agents because these make the use of the nerve stimulator ineffective. The patient is placed in a supine position with a shoulder roll to extend the neck. The head is turned away from the affected side and elevated to a 45-degree position to reduce venous congestion. The operative area is prepped and draped. The face is left exposed by placing a transparent dressing to allow facial movements to be observed during facial nerve stimulation.

INCISION   A preauricular incision is made starting at the upper end of the ear and passing vertically downward and then gently curving away from the angle of the mandible (Fig. 4–1A). The incision is continued anteriorly approximately two fingers-breadth below the inferior border of the mandible to avoid injury to the marginal mandibular branch of the facial nerve. To avoid capillary oozing, the skin can be infiltrated with 1% lidocaine with epinephrine.

PROCEDURE   The anterior flap is created in the subplatysmal plane close to the parotid fascia. Mobilization of the flap should not proceed beyond the anterior border of the parotid gland to avoid injury to the terminal branches of the facial nerve, because they lie in very superficial positions.

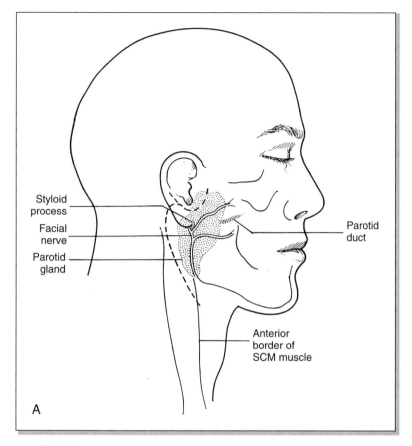

Styloid process

Facial nerve

Parotid gland

Parotid duct

Anterior border of SCM muscle

A

FIGURE 4–1 *A,* The incision used to perform parotidectomy.
Illustration continued on the following page

The posterior flap is elevated to expose the sternocleidomastoid muscle, the mastoid process, and the cartilage of the external auditory canal. To maintain exposure, the skin flaps can be sutured with 2-0 silk sutures to the drapes, and the earlobe should also be retracted superiorly using a 2-0 silk suture.

Posteriorly the lower border of the parotid gland is dissected off the sternocleidomastoid muscle. The following two structures are encountered: (1) the external jugular vein, which is divided and ligated with 2-0 silk sutures, and (2) the anterior branch of the greater auricular nerve that runs over the parotid gland, which is sacrificed. After these structures have been dealt with, the parotid gland is elevated until the anterior border of sternocleidomastoid muscle is identified. This dissection is continued cephalad toward the mastoid process. Deep to the sternocleidomastoid, the posterior belly of the digastric muscle is exposed. Using a fine Halsted mosquito clamp, the operator develops a plane of dissection between the gland and the cartilaginous part of the external auditory meatus until the bony part is reached. This dissection is continued superiorly as far as the zygomatic process of the temporal bone. Once the posterior dissection is complete, the parotid gland can be retracted forward and outward to begin identification of the facial nerve.

First, the V-shaped sulcus between the mastoid process and the cartilaginous part of the external auditory meatus is felt. Next, the tympanoparotid fascia will be encountered; this extends between the tympanomastoid fissure and the parotid gland. This fascia is elevated and divided with a scalpel. Approximately 1 cm anterior to the apex of this V-shaped sulcus, the facial nerve should be sought at the depth of the posterior belly of the digastric muscle (Fig. 4–1B). At this point the facial nerve is identified coursing forward toward the parotid gland and is less deeply placed, thus simplifying its exposure. A small artery, always encountered just superficial to the trunk of the facial nerve, requires ligation because it can bleed vigorously. Damage to the nerve is prevented if meticulous blunt dissection is directed in the axis of the nerve.

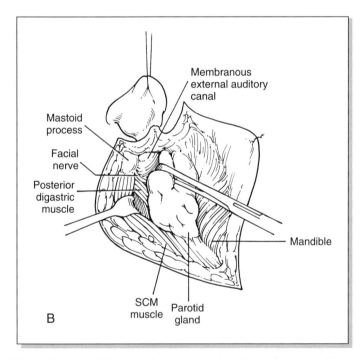

FIGURE 4–1 *Continued. B,* The cartilaginous part of the external auditory meatus is identified in relation to the mastoid process. The facial nerve is found at the depth of the posterior belly of the digastric muscle coursing forward toward the parotid gland. SCM, sternocleidomastoid.

After the trunk of the seventh nerve has been isolated, dissection proceeds forward in the plane of its branches. If dissection is carried only along the branches, several tunnels will be created but the bulk of the superficial lobe will remain unelevated. Instead, we prefer to create a plane just superficial to the branches. While keeping these branches under view, fine blunt hemostats are passed through the parotid gland at a right angle to the axis of the branch. The tissue is divided with bipolar forceps to avoid heat injury to the facial nerve branches. Use of bipolar electrocautery also avoids the troublesome bleeding that occurs when the parotid parenchyma is divided. Any vessel greater than 2 mm in diameter is ligated in continuity with 3-0 silk sutures and divided. If a dry field is maintained, the nerve is less likely to be inadvertently damaged. The gland is thus sequentially elevated off all the branches of the facial nerve. At the anterior border of the superficial lobe, the parotid duct (Stensen's duct) is identified, divided, and ligated. The superficial lobe is removed, and any persistent bleeding is controlled with bipolar electrocautery or fine ligatures.

If the deep lobe of the parotid gland also needs to be removed, several vascular structures first need to be secured. At the lower border of the deep portion of the parotid gland, the posterior facial vein is isolated, divided, and ligated with 2-0 silk sutures. Next, the posterior facial vein is separated from the marginal mandibular nerve before it is divided and ligated with 2-0 silk sutures. The lower border of the gland is elevated; deep to the posterior belly of the digastric muscle, the external carotid artery is divided and ligated. Posteriorly, the superficial temporal vessels are divided. At the anterior border of the gland, the internal maxillary and transverse facial vessels are divided. The individual branches of the facial nerve are dissected free from the parotid gland and retracted gently with either nerve hooks or vessel loops. The deep lobe is removed from the space between the divisions of the facial nerve or from below the lowermost division.

CLOSURE   A small 7-mm Jackson-Pratt drain is placed through a separate stab incision. The platysma is approximated with 3-0 absorbable sutures. The skin is closed with subcuticular 4-0 absorbable sutures. The closure can be reinforced with Steri-Strips.

CHAPTER 5

Submandibular Gland Resection

EMBRYOLOGY   The paired submandibular glands develop from the buds in the floor of the primitive mouth that grow on the lateral aspect of the tongue. The buds initially give rise to cords that canalize into ducts, and their ends differentiate into the acinar structures.

ANATOMY   The submandibular gland is located in the floor of the mouth and consists of a larger superficial part that communicates with a smaller deep part around the posterior border of the mylohyoid. The superficial part primarily lies within the digastric triangle and is bounded superomedially by the mylohyoid muscle, superolaterally by the mandible, and inferiorly by the skin platysma and investing layer of the deep cervical fascia. The facial artery is related to the posterior surface of the submandibular gland.

The deep part of the submandibular gland is located in the interval between the mylohyoid and the hyoglossus muscle. Emerging from the deep part of the gland is the submandibular duct (Wharton's duct), which opens at the base of the frenulum in the floor of the mouth. Other important structures that lie in the vicinity of the deep part of the submandibular gland are the lingual nerve, the submandibular ganglion superiorly, and the hypoglossal nerve inferiorly.

The blood supply of the submandibular gland is through branches of the facial and lingual arteries, and the venous drainage follows the respective facial and lingual veins.

The parasympathetic secretomotor supply is from the superior salivary nucleus of the seventh cranial nerve. These fibers reach the submandibular ganglion via the chorda tympani and submandibular ganglion.

PREOPERATIVE PREPARATION   Apart from basic investigations, the imaging studies of the submandibular gland, particularly plain radiograph of the floor of the mouth, sialogram for recurrent submandibular gland enlargement, or computed tomography of the neck for a solitary mass within the submandibular gland, are reviewed. Although indication for resection of the submandibular gland is usually based on clinical suspicion, results of fine-needle aspiration cytology, if performed, should be reviewed. Preoperatively the surgeon must determine by physical examination whether the hypoglossal, lingual, and marginal mandibular branches of the facial nerve are intact. Informed consent is obtained after the patient is informed about the risks of damage to the hypoglossal nerve, the lingual nerve, and the marginal mandibular branch of the facial nerve.

Operative Procedure

POSITION   The patient undergoes general anesthesia with endotracheal intubation, but anesthesiologists must refrain from using paralyzing agents because these may make the use of the nerve stimulator ineffective. The patient is placed in a supine position with a shoulder roll to extend the neck. The head is turned away from the affected side and elevated to a 45-degree position to reduce venous congestion. The operative area is prepped and draped. The face is left exposed by placing a transparent dressing to allow facial movements to be observed during facial nerve stimulation.

INCISION   An incision about 2 cm below and parallel to the body of the mandible is marked with an indelible pen (Fig. 5–1A). The skin is infiltrated with 1% lidocaine with epinephrine to avoid bleeding from the skin. The skin is incised with a no. 15 scalpel.

EXPOSURE AND OPERATIVE TECHNIQUE   The dermis is divided with cutting electrocautery down to the level of the platysma. In line with the incision, the platysma is also divided, and then superior and inferior flaps are created in the subplatysmal plane. Superiorly, the surgeon should be cognizant of the presence of the marginal mandibular branch of the facial nerve. The facial artery and vein will be encountered running deep to this nerve, and they are divided and ligated. In fact, retracting these vessels upward will protect the marginal mandibular branch of the facial nerve during subsequent dissection (Hayes-Martin maneuver). The superior border of the gland is freed from the body of the mandible.

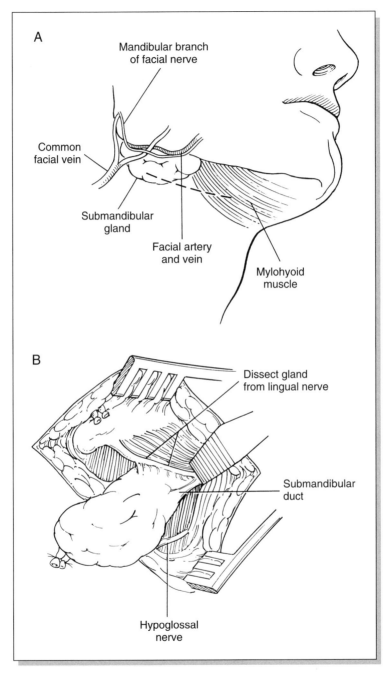

FIGURE 5-1 *A,* Incision used to perform submandibular gland resection. Important anatomic structures are shown. *B,* Mylohyoid muscle is retracted to expose the submandibular duct and lingual and hypoglossal nerves.

Dissection now proceeds toward the posterior aspect of the gland, and the posterior/common facial vein is exposed, isolated, divided, and ligated. Posteriorly, the gland is carefully elevated off the surface of the sternocleidomastoid muscle. Retracting the anterior border of the sternocleidomastoid muscle will expose the tortuous facial artery, which is ligated again. The superficial part of the submandibular gland is elevated from the underlying mylohyoid muscle. The posterior border of the mylohyoid muscle is identified and then retracted anteriorly with a loop retractor. This should expose the deep part of the submandibular gland and the important adjacent structures (Fig. 5–1*B*). These include the lingual nerve above and the hypoglossal nerve below.

Superiorly the branches from the lingual nerve to the submandibular ganglion are seen and divided. This allows the lingual nerve to retract superiorly and thus avoids injury. Next, the hypoglossal nerve, which will be seen emerging from beneath the anterior belly of the digastric muscle, is identified. The gland now remains attached only by its submandibular duct (Wharton's duct), lying between the lingual and hypoglossal nerves. The submandibular duct is clamped, divided, and ligated with 2-0 absorbable sutures. The operative area is inspected for hemostasis, and the retracted marginal mandibular nerve is returned to its normal position.

CLOSURE A 7-mm Jackson-Pratt drain is placed in the operative field. The platysma is approximated, with care taken not to entrap the already preserved marginal mandibular nerve. The skin is closed with 5-0 absorbable sutures.

CHAPTER 6

Radical and Modified Radical Neck Dissection

Operative Procedure

Radical Neck Dissection

POSITION The procedure is performed with the patient under general anesthesia with endotracheal intubation. The neck is extended by placing a rolled sheet beneath the shoulder. The head is rotated toward the opposite side. The patient is placed in the reverse Trendelenburg position, which aids in reducing the venous pressure.

INCISION Several incisions have been described in the literature, and the type used will depend on the preference of the surgeon. We have used the hockey-stick incision, which commences at the mastoid process, runs obliquely downward along the anterior border of the sternocleidomastoid muscle, and gently curves into a horizontal limb.

EXPOSURE AND OPERATIVE TECHNIQUE The incision is carried through the subcutaneous tissue, and the platysma is identified. The platysma is divided down to the enveloping layer of the deep cervical fascia. To facilitate creation of the flaps, the assistant can use skin hooks to retract the skin upward. While counter-traction is applied, the superior flap is elevated in the subplatysmal plane to the level of the mandible. Approximately 1 to 1.5 cm below the lower border of the body of the mandible, the mandibular branch of the facial nerve is identified. The greater auricular nerve is identified and preserved by dissecting superficially to the nerve. Superiorly where the platysma thins out, the plane of dissection is kept on the surface of the sternocleidomastoid muscle. The posterior flap is elevated until the anterior border of the trapezius muscle is identified. The dissection proceeds inferiorly to the clavicle and medially to the midline.

Posterior triangle dissection is started by skeletonizing the full length of the anterior border of the trapezius. Along the lower half of the trapezius the spinal accessory nerve is identified and transected. The free edge of the areolar tissue is grasped with multiple clamps to allow the assistant to provide upward retraction while it is elevated from the floor of the posterior triangle. The splenius capitis, levator scapulae, and scalenus medius are exposed (Fig. 6–1A). As medial dissection is continued, the sensory and motor roots of C2 and C3 will be encountered. The sensory roots are divided, and the motor roots are preserved. Further distal dissection deep to the sternocleidomastoid muscle should be avoided because the phrenic nerve can be injured.

Next, at the base of the posterior triangle the transverse cervical vessels are isolated, ligated, and divided. The inferior belly of the omohyoid muscle is identified, clamped, and divided. The heavy clamp is left on the proximal end of the omohyoid muscle to facilitate further dissection. Finally, the fibroadipose tissue containing lymphatics above the clavicle (base of posterior triangle) is carefully clamped, divided, and ligated. The external jugular vein is divided and ligated.

The sternal and clavicular attachments of the sternocleidomastoid muscle are divided carefully, thus exposing the carotid sheath. Beneath it the distal end of the internal jugular vein will be seen and is also dissected, after it is ensured that the vagus nerve is not adherent. The internal jugular vein is ligated in continuity with 2-0 silk sutures and transected. A transfixion 3-0 silk suture is placed on the distal stump. The specimen is retracted upward, and dissection is carefully undertaken along the carotid artery with a scalpel or electrocautery (Fig. 6–1B). The phrenic nerve will be seen lying on the surface of the anterior scalene muscle. As dissection proceeds cranially, it is also freed in the midline.

Now, the tissue in the submental area is dissected and elevated until the entire mylohyoid muscle is exposed. The lateral border of the muscle mylohyoid is retracted anteriorly to expose the critical structures within the submandibular triangle. Superiorly the lingual nerve will be identified with a branch to the submandibular gland. This branch is divided, which allows the lingual nerve to retract superiorly. Next, the hypoglossal nerve is identified as it is emerging from beneath the anterior belly of the digastric muscle. Between the two nerves will be the submandibular duct of

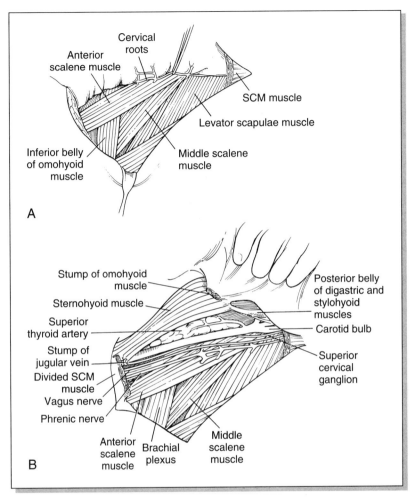

FIGURE 6–1 *A*, The muscles of the posterior triangle and the cervical sensory and motor roots are exposed. SCM, Sternocleidomastoid. *B*, The internal jugular vein has been divided and the specimen is carefully freed from the carotid sheath. Dissection is proceeding toward level I.

Wharton, which is clamped, divided, and ligated with 2-0 absorbable sutures. The submandibular gland can thus be elevated and can then be released by dividing the facial vessels present at its posterior border. This portion of the dissection is completed by elevating the rest of the lymphoareolar tissue off the posterior belly of the digastric muscle. The lower pole of the parotid gland is removed, which facilitates visualization of the upper end of the internal jugular vein. The operative field after completion of the procedure is shown in Figure 6–2.

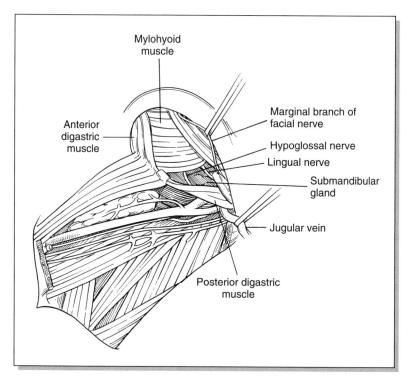

FIGURE 6–2 Operative field at completion of procedure.

CLOSURE Jackson-Pratt drains are placed. The platysma is carefully approximated with interrupted 3-0 absorbable sutures, and the skin is closed with subcuticular 4-0 absorbable sutures.

Modified Radical Neck Dissection

The position, incision, and flap elevation are similar to that described for radical neck dissection. When modified neck dissection is performed, either all or some of the following anatomic structures are preserved: sternocleidomastoid muscle, internal jugular vein, and spinal accessory nerve.

After the flaps are created, the spinal accessory nerve is identified at the anterior border of the trapezius and carefully freed along its course in the posterior triangle. The lymphoareolar tissue in the superior half of the posterior triangle is dissected from the underlying muscles and delivered beneath the previously identified spinal accessory nerve. The inferior half of level V is then completed, the inferior belly of the omohyoid muscle is divided, and the brachial plexus is exposed. With the specimen elevated, the cervical plexus comes into view. The cutaneous branches of the cervical plexus are divided, carefully preserving the motor nerve supply to the muscles of the posterior triangle and the contributions to the phrenic nerve.

Next, the fascia along the posterior border of the sternocleidomastoid muscle is incised along its entire length, and the muscle is completely freed from its fascial coverings. A Penrose drain is used to lift the sternocleidomastoid muscle. While the internal jugular vein is preserved, the contents of the carotid sheath are dissected upward toward the jugulodigastric area. The contents of the submandibular triangle are dissected in the usual fashion. Jackson-Pratt drains are placed, the platysma is approximated, and the skin is closed as described for radical neck dissection.

Thoracic Surgery

CHAPTER 7

Thoracotomy and Lung Resection

EMBRYOLOGY   The respiratory system begins as an entodermal outgrowth from the ventral surface of the foregut, immediately inferior to the hypobranchial eminence. This diverticulum begins to grow caudad to form the midline trachea and at its most distal portion divides into two lateral branches, the lung buds. The right lung bud divides into three branches, forming the main bronchi, and the left divides into two main branches, thus representing the adult pulmonary lobar anatomy. During this period, the respiratory diverticulum has a wide-open connection to the foregut that begins to separate due to the formation of the tracheoesophageal septum. The connection to the foregut is maintained only at the most proximal portion—the laryngeal orifice.

The lung buds are surrounded by splanchnic mesoderm, which forms the visceral pleura. As the lung buds further develop and repeatedly divide in a dichotomous fashion, they grow into the pericardioperitoneal canal. At the end of the sixth month, approximately 17 generations of subdivisions have formed, and at the seventh month the terminal bronchioli expand to form the alveoli. The block of mesodermal tissue surrounding the bronchial tree differentiates into cartilage, muscle, and blood vessels.

ANATOMY   The lungs are paired organs that lie within their pleural sacs and are attached to the mediastinum at the hilum. The lungs are spongy and elastic in consistency, which allows them to conform to the contours of the thoracic cavity. Each lung has an apex directed toward the thoracic inlet and a base lying on the diaphragm. The lungs are divided into lobes by fissures, which extend deep into their parenchyma. The oblique fissure divides the left lung into an upper lobe and a lower lobe. The oblique and horizontal fissures divide the right lung into upper, middle, and lower lobes. The anteroinferior part of the left upper lobe, lying adjacent to the cardiac notch, is known as the lingula and represents the middle lobe. However, there can be variations in the lobar pattern; in particular, the horizontal fissure may be incomplete and occasionally additional lobes may be present.

The trachea divides into the right and left main-stem bronchi. The left upper lobe bronchus arises from the main-stem bronchus within the lung and divides into five segmental bronchi, with two passing to the lingula. The left main-stem bronchus continues into the lower lobe and divides into five segmental branches. The right upper lobe bronchus arises from the right main-stem bronchus, and soon after entering the lung it divides into three segmental bronchi. The middle lobe divides into two segmental branches. Finally, the continuation of the right main-stem bronchus passes to the lower lobe and divides into five segmental branches. Each segmental bronchus is distributed to a functionally independent unit of lung tissue— a *bronchopulmonary segment*.

The bronchial branches of the descending thoracic aorta supply the lung. The bronchial veins drain into the azygos and hemiazygos veins. Lymphatic drainage is via the superficial subpleural lymphatic plexus and a deep plexus of vessels accompanying the bronchi. Both groups drain through hilar lymph nodes to the tracheobronchial nodes around the bifurcation of the trachea and then to the mediastinal lymphatic trunks. The pulmonary plexus provides the nerve supply to the lungs and contains the sympathetic fibers from the upper thoracic segments and the parasympathetic fibers from the vagus nerve.

PREOPERATIVE PREPARATION   Before any surgical intervention, the surgeon should review the chest x-ray, computed tomography scan of the chest, and results of the fiberoptic bronchoscopic biopsy. Positron emission tomography is now becoming the standard of care to assess for extrapulmonary metastases. Pulmonary function tests should have been obtained to determine whether the patient has adequate lung capacity to tolerate certain resections.

Operative Procedure

POSITION   For a standard posterolateral thoracotomy, the patient is placed in the straight lateral position. A Foley catheter, a central venous catheter on the side of the thoracotomy, and a radial artery catheter on the side opposite the thoracotomy are placed. General anesthesia is administered with the use of a double-lumen endobronchial tube. The patient is prepped and draped.

INCISION A posterolateral thoracotomy incision is made beginning posteriorly midway between the spinous process of the vertebrae and the medial border of the scapula, extends one to two fingers-breadth below the tip of the scapula, and is continued forward below the level of the nipple.

EXPOSURE AND OPERATIVE TECHNIQUE The incision is carried down to the level of the fascia. The auscultatory triangle is identified, and the fascia is divided to allow the surgeon to pass two fingers below the chest wall muscles (Fig. 7–1*A*). The latissimus dorsi posteriorly and the serratus anterior muscle anteriorly are divided with electrocautery (Fig. 7–1*B*). A scapula is lifted to count the ribs after the first or second rib is identified. The fifth intercostal space is chosen, and the intercostal muscles along the upper border of the sixth rib are divided with electrocautery (Fig. 7–1*C*). Before the surgeon enters the thoracic cavity, the ipsilateral lung is collapsed by the anesthesiologist to avoid injury. A careful exploration of the thoracic cavity is performed to inspect for presence of pleural implants, pleural effusion, and enlarged mediastinal lymph nodes. If the thoracotomy is for resection of a lung tumor, this lesion is identified and any extension of this lesion into the hilum or mediastinal structures is also defined. Dissection begins by opening the mediastinal pleura and carefully dissecting and identifying the main pulmonary artery and both the superior and inferior pulmonary veins. Vessel loops are placed around these vessels.

Right Pulmonary Resections

The initial step is to identify the azygos vein, which is ligated in continuity with 2-0 silk sutures and divided. Just inferior to the angle between the azygos vein and the superior vena cava, the main pulmonary artery can be located. Using a meticulous combination of sharp and blunt dissection, the operator places a vessel loop around the main pulmonary artery. Just inferior to the main pulmonary artery, the superior pulmonary vein is identified and carefully dissected, and a vessel loop is placed around it. More inferiorly, the inferior pulmonary ligament is carefully divided with Metzenbaum scissors or electrocautery. The inferior pulmonary vein is identified, and a vessel loop is placed around it.

Right Upper Lobectomy

To perform a right upper lobectomy, both the pulmonary artery and the vein are dissected peripherally toward the right upper lobe to carefully

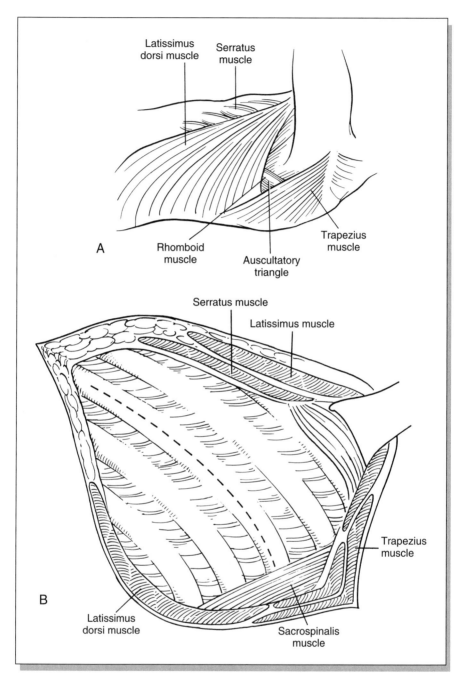

FIGURE 7–1 *A,* Muscles encountered when the thoracotomy incision is performed. The auscultatory triangle can be seen. *B,* Muscles have been divided, and the fifth rib is identified.

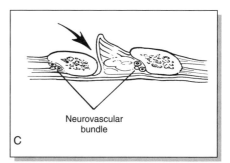

FIGURE 7–1 *Continued.* C, The fifth intercostal space is chosen and the intercostal muscles along the upper border of
the sixth rib are divided with electrocautery. The intercostal neurovascular
bundle can be seen beneath the lower
border of the rib.

Neurovascular
bundle

C

delineate the lobe's individual blood supply. First, the anterior and apico-
posterior segmental branches of the main pulmonary artery to the upper
lobe are ligated in continuity with 2-0 silk sutures, divided, and transfixed
proximally with 3-0 silk suture ligatures. Within the major fissure, the posterior segmental branch of the upper lobe is identified, ligated, transfixed,
and divided in a similar fashion. Within the minor fissure that exists
between the upper and middle lobes, the pulmonary venous drainage from
the upper lobe is identified and carefully dissected. The vein is ligated in continuity with 0 silk sutures, transfixed with 2-0 silk suture, and divided. At
this point, the lung is retracted forward to gain access to the posteriorly
placed bronchus. The right main-stem bronchus and the carina are identified. The upper lobe bronchus is identified and transected with a TA-30 stapler. In this fashion, the right upper lobectomy is completed.

Right Middle Lobectomy

For a right middle lobectomy, the pulmonary artery branch to the middle
lobe is identified, ligated with 0-0 silk sutures, transfixed with 2-0 silk
sutures, and divided. The middle lobe division of the superior pulmonary
vein is similarly ligated with 0-0 silk sutures, transfixed with 2-0 silk
sutures, and divided. With these two vessels addressed, the surgeon carefully
isolates the middle lobe bronchus and then transects it with a TA-30 stapler.

Right Lower Lobectomy

To perform a right lower lobectomy, the main pulmonary artery is followed
in the major fissure, and the segmental branches to the lower lobe are identified. The superior and basal segmental branches to the lower lobe are
carefully identified, ligated in continuity with 0 silk sutures, transfixed
with 2-0 silk sutures, and divided. Particular care is taken to avoid injury
to the middle lobe arteries. Next, attention is directed to the inferior pulmonary vein, where, after the surgeon has ensured that any drainage from
the middle lobe is protected, the inferior pulmonary vein is transected
with a TA-30 stapler. Again, within the same major fissure, the superior

segmental and the basal segmental bronchi are individually identified and transected with a TA-30 stapler.

Right Pneumonectomy

If the surgeon decides to perform a pneumonectomy to ensure complete resection of the tumor, this is fairly straightforward because dissection of all the primary vessels has already been performed. With the use of a TA-30 stapler, the pulmonary artery and then the superior and inferior pulmonary veins are transected. The lung is retracted anteriorly, and the right main-stem bronchus is carefully isolated and transected with a TA-30 stapler, taking care to avoid compromising the lumen of the left main-stem bronchus.

Left Lung Resection

After a thorough exploration of the left thoracic cavity is performed, the mediastinal pleura is carefully divided. After identification and preservation of the phrenic, vagal, and recurrent laryngeal nerves, the superior pulmonary artery and the superior and the inferior pulmonary veins are individually dissected and vessel loops are placed. To perform a lobectomy, the pulmonary artery is followed distally, which leads into the major fissure. The individual segmental branches of the pulmonary artery to the appropriate upper or lower lobe are carefully dissected, ligated in continuity with 0-0 silk sutures, and transfixed with 2-0 silk sutures. Alternatively, these vessels can be transected with either an endovascular stapler or a TA-30 stapler. Finally, the appropriate draining pulmonary vein is dissected and transected with a TA-30 stapler. With the pulmonary vein and the artery having been addressed, the underlying bronchus is exposed, which can be transected with a TA-30 stapler. If a left pneumonectomy is being performed, the pulmonary artery, pulmonary vein, and main-stem bronchus are stapled individually.

After the lung resection is completed, the lung is inflated and any leaks are closed with 3-0 or 4-0 absorbable sutures. Through two separate stab incisions, two chest tubes are inserted: One is directed to the apex (size 36 Fr) and the other toward the costophrenic sulcus (size 32 Fr curved). These are secured with 1-0 nonabsorbable sutures. The chest tubes are connected to a water seal and suction is applied.

CLOSURE The ribs are approximated with multiple pericostal 1-0 absorbable sutures. A Bailey rib approximator is helpful during the process of rib approximation. Latissimus dorsi and serratus anterior muscles are aligned and approximated with interrupted 2-0 silk sutures. The skin is approximated with staples.

CHAPTER 8

Ivor-Lewis Esophagectomy

EMBRYOLOGY   The esophagus is derived from the foregut and extends from the origin of the repiratory diverticulum to the primitive stomach. Elongation of the esophagus occurs due to the rapid growth of the body, particularly the adjacent lung and heart. The surrounding mesenchymal tissue forms the muscular covering of the esophagus.

ANATOMY   This is a tubular structure measuring 25 cm that begins just behind the cricoid cartilage at the level of the sixth cervical vertebra as a continuation of the pharynx. The upper end is approximately 15 cm from the incisors. The esophagus descends through the neck and posterior mediastinum to pass through the diaphragm at the level of T10 to join the stomach in the abdomen. In the neck, the esophagus lies anterior to the prevertebral fascia and posterior to the trachea, and in the groove between these structures lie the important recurrent laryngeal nerves. Laterally, the esophagus is related to the thyroid lobes and the carotid sheath.

Upon entering the thoracic cavity, the esophagus initially lies on the left side and is subsequently pushed to the midline by the aortic arch. The esophagus then crosses the midline and assumes a right-sided position within the right thoracic cavity. Before piercing the diaphragm, the esophagus is displaced toward the left and is found anterior to the descending thoracic aorta. Posteriorly and starting from above downward, it is related to the thoracic duct, the hemiazygos vein, the right posterior intercostal arteries, and finally the descending aorta. Below the trachea, the esophagus is crossed anteriorly by the left main-stem bronchus and then the pericardium, which separates it from the atrium. The mediastinum is present on the lateral aspect bilaterally. On the right side the azygos vein arches forward above the lung root. On the left side it is separated from the mediastinal pleura by the left subclavian artery, the thoracic duct, the aortic arch, and the descending aorta.

As the esophagus passes through the right crus of the diaphragm, it lies on the left of the midline. It is accompanied through the hiatus by the vagi (the left vagus lies anteriorly and the right vagus lies posteriorly) and lymphatics. The abdominal esophagus measures approximately 3 cm in length and is covered anterolaterally by the peritoneum. The left lateral lobe of the liver is present anteriorly.

The blood supply of the esophagus is as follows: upper one third, inferior thyroid artery; middle one third, descending thoracic aorta; and lower one third, left gastric artery. The respective venous drainage for the esophagus occurs via the inferior thyroid, azygos, and left gastric veins. Similarly, the lymphatic drainage from the upper third is to the deep cervical lymph nodes, from the middle third is to the posterior mediastinal lymph nodes, and from the distal third is to the celiac axis.

SPECIAL PREOPERATIVE PREPARATION Esophagectomy is commonly indicated for carcinoma of the esophagus. A preoperative barium swallow is performed. To accurately assess the extent and anatomic location of the tumor, an upper gastrointestinal endoscopy is performed. A computed tomography scan of the chest and upper abdomen is obtained to determine the extent of local invasion and presence of suspicious lymphadenopathy. If available, an endoscopic ultrasound may also be obtained because it allows an accurate determination of the depth of the tumor infiltration and also ascertains whether any suspicious paraesophageal or celiac lymphadenopathy is present. Biopsies are obtained, and pathologic diagnosis should be confirmed. For lesions in the mid-esophagus, a preoperative bronchoscopy is indicated to exclude invasion of the left main-stem bronchus or trachea. Preoperative cardiac evaluation, including an echocardiogram and Persantine thallium scan, should be performed. Pulmonary function tests should also be conducted.

Operative Procedure

POSITION The patient is placed in the supine position. An epidural catheter can be requested for postoperative pain management. The patient then undergoes general anesthesia with endotracheal intubation using a double-lumen tube. A nasogastric tube, Foley catheter, and sequential pneumatic compression devices are placed in the lower extremities. The abdomen, chest, and neck are prepped with Betadine and then draped with sterile drapes in the usual fashion.

Abdominal Portion

INCISION A midline incision is made from the xiphoid to below the umbilicus and extended down through the subcutaneous tissue to the linea alba (Fig. 8–1). The preperitoneal fat and peritoneum are opened using electrocautery. The ligamentum teres is divided between clamps and ligated with 2-0 silk sutures. The falciform ligament is divided to the level of the suprahepatic inferior vena cava. An upper hand retractor is useful at this stage to facilitate upward retraction of the right and left costal margins. A Balfour self-retaining retractor is also placed.

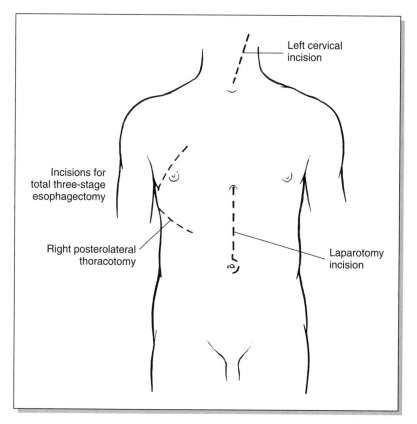

FIGURE 8–1 The incisions used to perform a total three-stage esophagectomy.

EXPOSURE AND OPERATIVE TECHNIQUE A thorough exploration of the abdomen is performed to evaluate the presence of metastatic disease in the liver, celiac axis lymph nodes, and peritoneal implants. In the absence of metastatic disease, the surgeon proceeds with an Ivor-Lewis esophagogastrectomy. The duodenum is mobilized by performing a wide Kocher maneuver. The key aspect of mobilizing the stomach and maintaining its viability is by dividing the greater omentum outside the gastroepiploic arcade, which must be kept intact (Fig. 8–2). Mobilization of the greater curvature of the stomach is begun approximately 6 to 8 cm proximal to the pylorus, where usually the clear area within the gastrocolic ligament is identified and incised to enter the lesser sac. Using the left hand at all times to palpate and preserve the gastroepiploic arcade, the operator divides the greater omentum along the greater curvature between clamps and ligates it with 2-0 silk sutures. If the omentum is very fatty, additional 3-0 silk transfixion suture ligatures are placed. This process of dividing the greater omentum is continued proximally until the left gastroepiploic artery is reached, and it

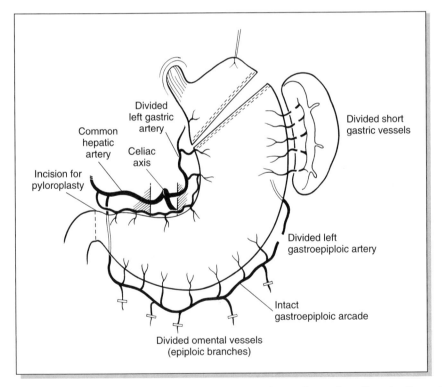

FIGURE 8–2 Key elements of the mobilization of the stomach, with retention of an intact gastroepiploic arcade, pyloroplasty, and division of the gastric cardia to create a gastric tube.

also is divided and ligated. To improve exposure of the short gastric vessels and avoid splenic injury, the spleen is displaced medially by placement of moist laparotomy pads in the left upper quadrant. The short gastric vessels are individually clamped with fine long Schnidt clamps, divided, and ligated with 2-0 silk sutures. The dissection is continued proximally over the gastric cardia, where the gastrophrenic ligament is divided with electrocautery. Next, with the stomach lifted upward, the left gastric vein is identified in the lesser sac, ligated in continuity with 0-0 silk suture ligatures, and suture ligated with a 2-0 silk transfixion sutures before division.

Next, the left gastric artery is carefully dissected, ligated, and divided in a similar fashion. Now attention is directed toward mobilizing the distal esophagus. Exposure of the esophageal hiatus is improved by sharply dividing the left triangular ligament of the liver. This allows retraction of the left lateral lobe of the liver. The peritoneum overlying the esophageal hiatus is incised, and the two diaphragmatic crura are visualized. Dissection is performed along the left and the right crura to remove all the paraesophageal fibrofatty tissue containing lymph nodes and incorporate it into the esophagus as an en bloc resection.

As the esophagus is freed circumferentially with the adjacent fibrofatty tissue, the vagal trunks are identified and transected, which further facilitates esophageal mobilization. The vagus nerves are secured with hemoclips before division to prevent bleeding from the accompanying vasa nervorum. Under direct vision the esophageal dissection is continued up into the posterior mediastinum. To facilitate this, the diaphragm can be separated from the pericardium and divided vertically. By now the duodenum, stomach, and esophagus have been completely mobilized. Because the vagal trunks have been divided, it is necessary to perform a pyloroplasty. The pylorus is identified, and 2-0 silk stay sutures are placed. A transverse incision is made across the first part of the duodenum, pylorus, and distal 2 to 2.5 cm of the stomach. This incision is closed in a longitudinal manner using a single layer of inverting 3-0 silk interrupted sutures (see Fig. 8–2). Alternatively, a two-layer closure, with an inner layer of continuous 3-0 absorbable sutures followed by an outer seromuscular layer of 3-0 silk interrupted Lembert sutures, may be performed. Finally, the ligament of Treitz is identified and an area distal to this is chosen for placement of a feeding jejunostomy. The abdominal cavity is irrigated and hemostasis achieved. The linea alba is closed using running continuous 1-0 polypropylene monofilament sutures. The skin is approximated with staples.

Thoracic Portion

The patient is turned on the left side and placed in the left lateral decubitus position to perform the right posterolateral thoracotomy. An axillary roll is placed, and the patient's position is sustained with the use of sand-bags and tape. The right chest is prepped and draped in the usual fashion. A right posterolateral thoracotomy incision is made, and dissection is continued down to the chest wall (see Fig. 8–1). Posteriorly, two sets of muscles, the trapezius superficially and deep to it the rhomboid major, are encountered and divided with electrocautery. Anteriorly, two additional muscles, the latissimus dorsi muscle superficially and deep to it the serratus anterior muscle, are encountered and divided in a similar fashion.

Before the surgeon enters the thoracic cavity, the anesthesiologist is requested to collapse the right lung. The thoracic cavity is entered through the fifth intercostal space, and a Finochietto rib retractor is placed. The lung is retracted superiorly and medially, and the inferior pulmonary ligament is transected. The esophagus is identified and fully mobilized within the mediastinum. A wide lymph node dissection extending from the arch of the aorta down to the esophageal hiatus is performed. All lymphatic tissue is cleared laterally and posteriorly off the aorta and medially off the area of the tracheobronchial tree as well as the inferior pulmonary veins. These lymph nodes are incorporated into the specimen. The azygos vein is identified, carefully dissected, ligated in continuity, and divided. Stay sutures using 0-0 silk are placed on each side of the esophagus, which is sharply transected. The stomach is pulled into the chest and, using a GIA-90 linear stapler, the proximal stomach is divided along the lesser curvature. The specimen is thus removed and sent to the pathologist to check margins by frozen section. If the margins show evidence of tumor, a total esophagectomy must be considered by extending the dissection into the cervical region (see below). If margins are clear, an end-to-side esophagogastric anastomosis is performed.

In preparation for the anastomosis, first the stomach is secured to the prevertebral fascia with a few interrupted 2-0 silk sutures. A two-layer anastomosis is performed by first placing the outer posterior layer of muscular sutures using 2-0 silk. Next, an inner suture line encompassing all layers is placed using 3-0 silk sutures. Finally, the anastomosis is completed with an anterior layer created by rolling the stomach up onto the esophagus using 2-0 silk interrupted Lembert sutures. The integrity of the anastomosis can be tested by injecting methylene blue into the nasogastric tube while occluding the stomach. The thoracic cavity is irrigated and two chest tubes are placed: a 36 Fr angled chest tube placed toward the costophrenic sulcus and a 32 Fr chest tube directed toward the apex. These are anchored in place with 0-0 nonabsorbable braided sutures.

CLOSURE   The thoracotomy incision is closed by approximating the ribs with several 1-0 chromic pericostal sutures. With the assistance of the Bailey rib approximator, the pericostal sutures are tied down. The divided muscles are approximated in layers with 0-0 absorbable sutures. The subcutaneous layers are approximated with running continuous 2-0 absorbable sutures. The skin is closed with staples. The chest tubes are connected to an underwater seal and placed on suction.

If a total esophagectomy needs to be performed to obtain a sufficient margin, the esophagogastric anastomosis has to be performed in the neck. In this case, the procedure expands to three stages.

Cervical Portion

In the original description of the three-stage esophagectomy by McKeown, access to the cervical esophagus was obtained from the right side of the neck. However, the dissection can also be performed from the left side of the neck. The patient's head is turned to the right, and an incision is made along the anterior border of the left sternocleidomastoid muscle; the lower end of the incision can be extended forward across he sternal notch if necessary. The incision is deepened through the subcutaneous tissue.

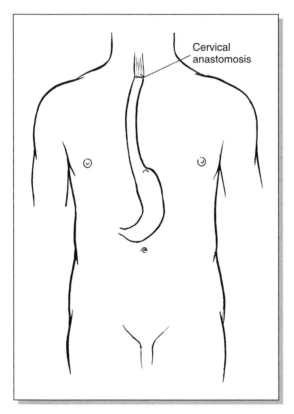

FIGURE 8-3 Completed cervical anastomosis.

The platysma is divided and a Weitlaner self-retaining retractor is placed. The middle thyroid vein is ligated in continuity with 3-0 silk sutures. The sternocleidomastoid muscle and the carotid sheath are retracted laterally, whereas the thyroid gland and the larynx are retracted medially. This exposes the inferior constrictor and the cervical esophagus. With blunt digital dissection, the esophagus is mobilized and the posterior mediastinum is entered. The presence of a nasogastric tube or the esophageal bougie facilitates the identification and dissection of the esophagus. To avoid injury to the recurrent laryngeal nerve, dissection should be performed close to the esophageal wall. The previously mobilized stomach and the thoracic esophagus are drawn up into the neck. The cardia is divided along the lesser curvature with a GIA-60 linear stapler. The cervical esophagus is divided, and the resected specimen is sent to pathology for margin assessment by frozen section. The fundus of the stomach is opened, and an end-to-end anastomosis is constructed as a single layer using 3-0 silk sutures (Fig. 8–3). Alternatively, a two-layer anastomosis can be performed with an outer layer of 3-0 silk and an inner layer of 3-0 absorbable sutures.

CLOSURE   The platysma is approximated with 3-0 absorbable sutures. The skin is closed with staples.

CHAPTER 9

Esophageal Perforation

ANATOMY AND EMBRYOLOGY   See Chapter 8.

PREOPERATIVE PREPARATION   Any clinical suspicion of esophageal perforation must be confirmed with imaging studies, such as chest and lateral cervical radiographs or Gastrografin swallow, to establish the presence and determine site and extent of the perforation. The patient should have nothing by mouth, intravenous fluid resuscitation is initiated, and broad-spectrum antibiotics are administered. The patient should be closely monitored; therefore, a Foley catheter is inserted and, if necessary, invasive hemodynamic monitoring such as a central venous or pulmonary artery catheter should be instituted.

The surgical approach depends on the location of perforation, etiology, and whether there has been a delay in presentation or diagnosis.

Operative Procedure

Perforation of Cervical Esophagus

POSITION   The patient is placed in the supine position with the head turned toward the right side. A log roll is placed beneath the shoulders to assist in extending the neck. The neck and the chest are prepped and draped in the usual manner.

INCISION   An oblique incision along the anterior border of the sternoclei-domastoid muscle is made with a no. 15 scalpel and extended from the angle of the mandible to the sternoclavicular junction (Fig. 9–1).

EXPOSURE AND OPERATIVE TECHNIQUE   The incision is carried through the subcutaneous tissues. The platysma is divided with electrocautery, and the fascia along the anterior border of the sternocleidomastoid muscle is similarly incised. The sternocleidomastoid muscle is retracted posteri-orly. Next, the superior belly of the omohyoid muscle, which crosses the operative field, is divided with electrocautery and ligated with 2-0 silk sutures. A Weitlaner retractor is placed for exposure. The carotid sheath is retracted laterally, whereas the strap muscles (sternohyoid and ster-nothyroid muscles) are retracted medially to expose the thyroid gland. The middle thyroid vein is ligated in continuity with 3-0 silk sutures and divided. The thyroid gland is carefully rotated medially to expose the inferior thyroid artery and the recurrent laryngeal nerve. At times it may be necessary to divide and ligate the inferior thyroid artery to improve exposure. The esophagus is identified and carefully dissected, and the site

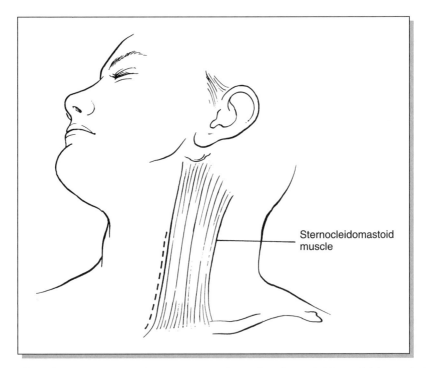

Sternocleidomastoid muscle

FIGURE 9–1   Incision along the anterior border of the sternocleidomastoid muscle to expose the cervical esophagus.

of perforation is located. The tissue around the perforation is carefully debrided and prepared for closure unless there is marked edema and inflammation due to delay in diagnosis. The mucosa is carefully approximated with interrupted 4-0 absorbable sutures. The muscular layer of the esophagus is approximated with 3-0 silk interrupted Lembert sutures (Fig. 9–2A). An adjacent viable muscle flap is constructed from the sternocleidomastoid muscle, and this is used to buttress the suture line and is secured with 3-0 silk sutures. The wound is carefully irrigated, and through a separate stab incision a Jackson-Pratt drain is placed in the retroesophageal space and secured with 3-0 monofilament sutures.

CLOSURE   The platysma is approximated with interrupted 3-0 absorbable sutures. The skin is approximated with staples.

Perforation of Thoracic Esophagus

POSITION   The patient is placed in either the left or the right lateral decubitus position, depending on the location of the perforation. The patient must be carefully secured and any areas of pressure padded. A double-lumen tube should be inserted by the anesthesiologists. To expose the upper esophagus and mid-esophagus, the right thoracic cavity is entered via a right posterolateral thoracotomy through the right fifth intercostal space. The lower half of the esophagus may be approached through a left posterolateral thoracotomy.

INCISION   The standard posterolateral thoracotomy incision is made, and the subcutaneous tissue is divided (see Chapter 7 for details). The latissimus dorsi and serratus anterior muscles are divided with electrocautery. The anesthesiologist is asked to collapse the ipsilateral lung, and the intercostal muscles and the pleura are divided to enter the thoracic cavity. The mediastinal pleura is incised, and any pleural fluid or purulent material should be cultured and evacuated. The esophagus is identified and carefully dissected circumferentially. A small Penrose drain is passed around it to facilitate retraction.

Once the site of the perforation is identified, it is carefully debrided unless there is marked edema due to inflammation that will prevent primary closure. A nasogastric tube is passed by the anesthesiologist. The mucosa is approximated with interrupted 3-0 absorbable sutures. The muscular layer is closed with interrupted 3-0 silk Lembert sutures (see Fig. 9–2A). To reinforce the closure, an adjacent rectangular pleural or an intercostal muscle flap is constructed. The flap is loosely wrapped around the esophagus and secured with multiple interrupted 3-0 silk sutures (Fig. 9–2B).

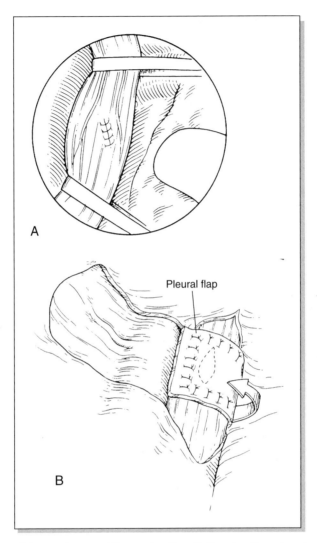

FIGURE 9–2 *A,* Primary closure of the perforation. *B,* Construction of a pleural flap.

On occasions when there has been considerable delay in presentation, the esophageal wall will be very edematous at exploration. One of the options involves closing the esophageal perforation over a T-tube. Alternatively, temporary esophageal exclusion and diversion can be performed. After the perforation is repaired with interrupted nonabsorbable 3-0 sutures, it is reinforced with an intercostal pedicle flap. Next, the esophagus is excluded by ligating it either with 2-0 chromic catgut sutures below the perforation deep to the vagus nerve or, much less frequently, with a TA-55 stapler containing absorbable staples. The staples are absorbed and the lumen becomes reestablished in 3 weeks. Proximal diversion is accomplished by creating a cervical esophagostomy. An oblique incision is made along the anterior border of the sternocleidomastoid muscle, and dissection proceeds as described in the earlier section on perforation of the cervical esophagus. The cervical esophagus is identified and carefully mobilized. A longitudinal incision is made on the lateral aspect of the esophageal wall, and the incision is sutured to the skin with 4-0 absorbable sutures. Alternatively, an 18 Fr Salem sump tube is placed via a cervical esophagostomy and secured with a double purse-string 2-0 or 3-0 absorbable suture and nonabsorbable sutures. The sump tube is brought out via a separate stab incision in the skin and placed on suction. A decompression gastrostomy and a feeding jejunostomy are placed. In most situations, it is preferable to attempt closure of the perforation with flap reconstruction and wide drainage rather than any exclusion technique. Finally, the thoracic cavity is irrigated.

CLOSURE   Two chest tubes are placed, an angled 32 Fr directed toward the costophrenic sulcus and a straight 36 Fr placed at the level of the esophageal closure. The lung is inflated. The ribs are approximated with several 0-0 chromic pericostal sutures or other absorbable sutures. The latissimus dorsi and serratus anterior muscles are approximated with continuous 2-0 absorbable sutures. The skin is approximated with staples. The chest tubes are secured with 0-0 nonabsorbable sutures. If the neck and the abdominal cavity have been opened, these are closed in the usual fashion. The gastrostomy and jejunostomy tubes are secured with 3-0 monofilament sutures.

Perforation of Abdominal Esophagus

POSITION   The patient is placed in the supine position.

INCISION   A midline incision extending from the xiphoid to just below the umbilicus is made.

EXPOSURE AND OPERATIVE TECHNIQUE   The linea alba is incised and the peritoneal cavity entered. Any fluid in the upper abdomen is cultured and suctioned. The peritoneal reflection over the esophageal hiatus is incised to expose the two diaphragmatic crura. With careful blunt digital dissection, the esophagus is encircled and a Penrose drain is placed for traction. The left triangular ligament of the liver may be divided and the left lateral lobe is retracted if additional exposure is required. The area of the perforation is located, devitalized tissue is debrided, and the area is prepared for closure. Usually two nasogastric tubes are inserted by the anesthesiologist and directed under vision into the stomach. This is done to avoid narrowing of the esophageal lumen during the repair. The mucosa is carefully approximated with interrupted 3-0 or 4-0 absorbable sutures. The muscular layer of the esophagus is approximated with 3-0 silk interrupted Lembert sutures. The primary repair can be buttressed with a diaphragmatic pedicle flap or omental onlay graft. Alternatively, the adjacent fundus may be used to buttress the closure. For this the gastric fundus is mobilized by dividing the esophagophrenic ligament. After completion of the procedure, one of the nasogastric tubes is removed. A Jackson-Pratt drain is placed near the hiatus. Finally, a feeding jejunostomy is placed.

CLOSURE The abdomen is closed in the standard fashion.

Breast Surgery

CHAPTER 10

Breast Biopsy

Operative Procedure

POSITION   The patient lies in the supine position with the ipsi-lateral arm abducted to 90 degrees. The entire breast is prepped, and sterile drapes are placed. The procedure may be performed under general anesthesia or under local anesthesia with accompanying sedation provided by the anesthesiologist.

INCISION   A curvilinear incision is marked directly over a palpable mass. A circumareolar incision can be used for central lesions. The incision should be planned appropriately so that it can be incorporated in subsequent mastectomy if needed. Avoid linear radial incisions. The incision should be long enough to allow the mass to be removed easily without excessive skin retraction.

EXPOSURE AND OPERATIVE TECHNIQUE   The steps involved in performing the breast biopsy are outlined in Figure 10–1. The skin and subcutaneous tissue are infiltrated with 1% lidocaine and incised. Additional local anesthesia is injected within the adjacent breast tissue. Breast flaps are created using sharp dissection. Dissection proceeds while aiming to achieve at least a 1-cm margin around the breast mass.

   The mass with the accompanying breast tissue is grasped and retracted toward the surgeon while counter-traction is provided with a deep Richardson retractor. The mass is sharply dissected circumferentially until the breast tissue can be lifted out of the wound. The specimen is excised after ensuring that adequately deep margins

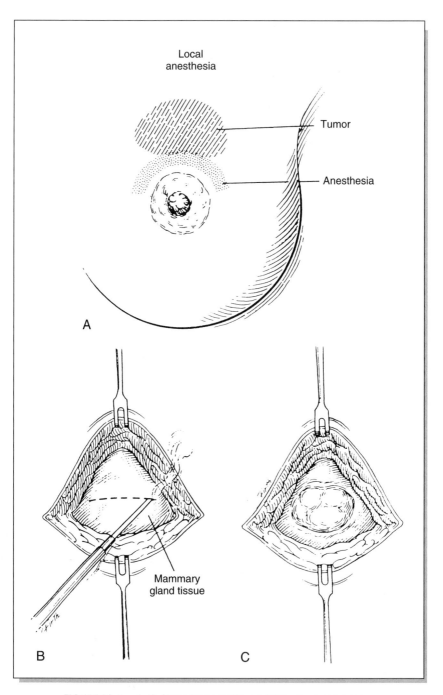

Local
anesthesia

Tumor

Anesthesia

A

Mammary
gland tissue

B   C

FIGURE 10–1 *A–C,* Steps involved in excision of a breast mass.

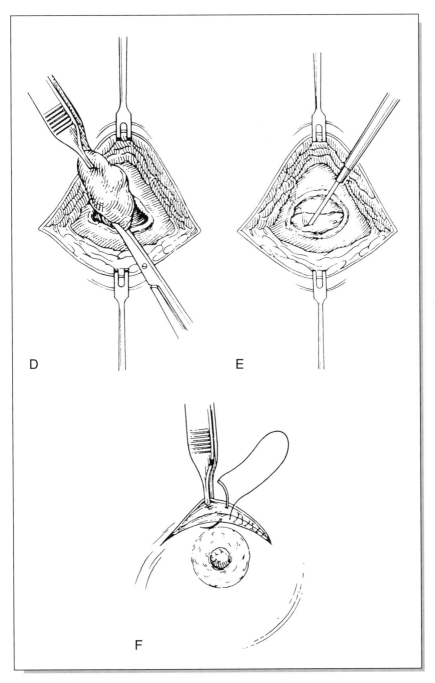

FIGURE 10–1 *Continued.* *D–F,* Steps involved in excision of a breast mass.

have been achieved. The specimen should be oriented for the pathologist by placing a single short suture at the superior margin and a long suture at the lateral margin. The pathologist should be requested to examine the specimen and determine if gross margins have been obtained. Further breast tissue can be removed in areas with close margins.

For mammographically detected nonpalpable lesions, preoperative needle localization is performed by the radiologist (see Fig. 10–1A). The two views of the mammogram (craniocaudal and mediolateral) are examined to determine the location of the mammographic lesion in relation to the needle. The nipple shadow is used as a reference point to ascertain the location of the needle tip within the breast. The location of the mammographic lesion can be estimated in relation to the skin entry site of the localizing wire. An attempt is made to place the skin incision directly over the lesion to avoid tunneling during the biopsy. A curvilinear skin incision should be made, then breast flaps should be created for a short distance. The wire is pulled out of the skin so that it emerges out of the incision. Manipulation of the needle should be minimized to improve success of excising the mammographic index lesion. Dissection proceeds along the axis of the needle. Adequate breast tissue should be excised in the region of the lesion to ensure that sufficient margins have been obtained. The resected specimen is sent for radiography to determine if the mammographic lesion has been successfully removed. Any close margins require further excision of breast tissue. The specimen is appropriately oriented for the pathologist. The breast cavity is irrigated, and hemostasis is achieved. If the biopsy is being performed for breast cancer, the edge of the cavity is delineated with hemoclips. This assists the radiation oncologist in providing postoperative radiation therapy. Drainage of the breast cavity or reapproximation of the breast tissue is not performed.

CLOSURE   The dermis is approximated with interrupted 3-0 absorbable sutures, and the skin is closed with subcuticular 4-0 absorbable sutures and reinforced with Steri-Strips.

CHAPTER 11

Modified Radical and Total Mastectomy

EMBRYOLOGY At 6 weeks' gestation a thickened strip of ectoderm, called the "mammary ridge," develops and extends from the base of the forelimb to the proximal part of the hindlimb. A small segment of this ridge persisting in the thoracic area penetrates the underlying mesenchymal tissue and proliferates to form multiple lactiferous ducts. Secondary buddings give rise to smaller ducts and alveolar tissue. The surrounding adipose and fibrous tissues are derived from the mesenchyme. A small pit forms in the epidermis and ultimately develops into the nipple–areola complex. Fragments of the epidermal tissue persisting along the "mammary line" can lead to accessory nipples.

ANATOMY The breast consists of glandular tissue that lies within the superficial fascia of the anterior chest wall. The base of the breast extends from the second rib to the sixth rib and from the lateral edge of the sternum to the midaxillary line. Breast tissue lies superficial to the deep fascia (pectoralis fascia), except for the axillary tail of Spence. This is a prolongation of breast tissue from its upper outer aspect, which passes up to the level of the third rib in the axilla. It enters the axilla through an opening in the axillary fascia known as the foramen of Langer. Thus, the axillary tail is the only segment of the breast that lies deep to the deep fascia.

The breast is anchored to the overlying skin and to the underlying pectoral fascia by fibrous bands known as Cooper's ligaments. The breast tissue is composed of numerous alveoli that make up lobules, which aggregate such that their ducts pass toward the nipple–areola complex. The ducts dilate into an ampulla just before their termination on the nipple.

The blood supply of the breast is derived from (1) perforating branches of the internal thoracic (mammary) artery to the second, third, and fourth intercostal spaces; (2) branches of the lateral thoracic artery, which is a branch originating from the second part of the axillary artery; and (3) lateral branches of the intercostal arteries to the second, third, and fourth intercostal arteries. The venous drainage corresponds to that of the arteries.

Knowledge of the lymphatic drainage of the breast is important in management of breast carcinoma. The subcutaneous subareolar plexus of Sappey and the submammary plexus in the fascia covering the pectoralis major muscle are not important in the lymph drainage of breast parenchyma. Lymphatics arising in the lobules pass through the breast parenchyma and the axillary tail of Spence and drain mainly into the anterior axillary/pectoral nodes. Some drain into the posterior group and then pass to the central and apical groups. Thus, the axillary nodes receive approximately 75% of the lymphatic drainage of the breast. Parasternal nodes along the internal mammary vessels may receive lymph from both the medial and lateral aspects of the breast. The lymphatic drainage of the skin over the breast is as follows: Outer aspects drain to the axillary nodes, upper quadrants drain to the supraclavicular nodes, and the inner part drains to the internal mammary chain. Furthermore, the lymphatics of the skin can cross the midline to communicate with the plexus of the opposite breast.

The anatomy of the axilla is discussed separately in Chapter 12.

SPECIAL PREOPERATIVE PREPARATION   The patient undergoes a thorough history and physical with special reference to the cardiopulmonary system. Routine laboratory tests are ordered. Review of the following investigations is necessary before the operation:

1. Histology of the breast lesion, which may have been obtained by fine-needle aspiration, core biopsy, or excisional biopsy.

2. Mammogram to evaluate whether the malignancy is multifocal or multicentric, because these issues are important when discussing surgical options.

3. Ultrasonography or computed tomography of the liver if metastasis is suspected.

4. Computed tomography of the chest if any abnormality is noted on the chest radiograph.

Informed consent is obtained after all the surgical options have been discussed with the patient. If there is concern regarding reconstruction, the patient should be evaluated by a plastic surgeon preoperatively. A decision can then be made regarding immediate or delayed reconstruction according to the preference of the patient.

Operative Procedure

POSITION The patient is placed in the supine position with the ipsilateral arm abducted at 90 degrees. The patient undergoes general anesthesia and endotracheal intubation. The axilla is shaved. The skin is prepped and draped from the neck down to the costal margin, including the ipsilateral arm. The surgeon stands on the side of the mastectomy to be performed, with the first assistant on the opposite side. The second assistant stands on the anesthetic side of the arm board.

INCISION A transverse elliptic incision with a 3-cm clearance around the tumor is outlined with an indelible pen. The incision extends from the lateral edge of the sternum medially to the midaxillary line laterally (Fig. 11–1). Note, however, that the incision should be below the axillary hairline.

EXPOSURE AND OPERATIVE TECHNIQUE The skin is incised until the subcutaneous tissue is identified. Dissecting any deeper at this point is avoided because it can lead to the development of false planes during creation of flaps. Several Adair clamps are placed along the upper incision at about 5-cm intervals to provide vertical traction by the assistant. Using a laparotomy pad, counter-traction is applied on the breast in the caudal direction. To avoid entry into the incorrect plane, the dermis is carefully freed from the underlying subcutaneous tissue. As downward traction is applied to the breast, Cooper's ligaments will come into view. The superior flap is created by dividing Cooper's ligaments extending between the superficial fascia of the breast and the subdermal adipose tissue. If the correct plane is entered, minimal bleeding should be encountered. The upper limit of the dissection is at the level of the clavicle. The pectoralis major fascia is identified from the medial margin to the lateral edge of the pectoralis major muscle. Once the upper flap is created, it should be covered with a moist laparotomy pad. Using the same technique described above, the inferior flap is created. The inferior flap extends down to the rectus sheath from the fifth rib medially to the latissimus dorsi laterally. The overall limits of the dissection include the clavicle superiorly, the lateral sternal edge medially, the latissimus dorsi muscle laterally, and the rectus sheath inferiorly (see Fig. 11–1).

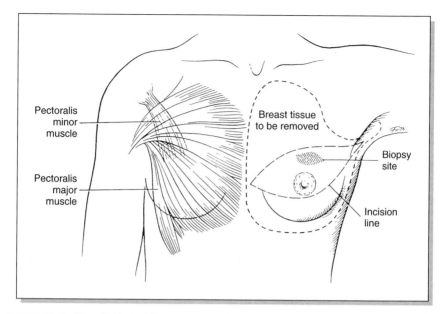

FIGURE 11–1 The elliptic incision encompassing the prior biopsy site and the limits of dissection are shown. The underlying muscles are seen on the left. (Redrawn from Hindle WH. Breast care: A clinical guidebook for women's primary health care providers. New York: Springer-Verlag, 1999.)

As the upper flap is retracted with medium-sized Richardson retractors, the pectoral fascia is incised, and the breast tissue is dissected off the underlying pectoralis major muscle using sharp dissection (Fig. 11–2). The pectoralis fascia is included with the specimen. Because the breast tissue is more adherent near the sternum, this dissection should be started from the lateral aspect and extended in the medial direction. Once the breast tissue is freed near the lateral sternal edge, dissection is continued until the lateral edge of the pectoralis major muscle is identified. The lateral edge is clearly delineated with sharp dissection. Further dissection from this point on differs, depending on whether a total or a modified radical mastectomy is to be performed. If a total mastectomy is being performed, the axillary tail is resected but the lymphatic tissue is left undisturbed. However, if a modified radical mastectomy is being performed, attention is now directed toward performing the axillary dissection.

Axillary Dissection Once the lateral edge of the pectoralis major muscle is dissected free, it is retracted upward with two right-angle retractors. This exposes the interpectoral fat and Rotter nodes. The interpectoral fat, which needs to be included in the specimen, is sharply dissected with Metzenbaum scissors to skeletonize the underlying pectoralis minor muscle. The lateral pectoral nerve and vessels lying along the medial

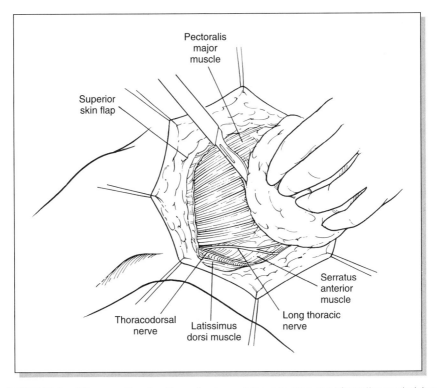

Pectoralis
major
muscle

Superior
skin flap

Serratus
anterior
muscle

Long thoracic
nerve

Thoracodorsal
nerve

Latissimus
dorsi muscle

FIGURE 11–2 After creating the flaps, the breast tissue is dissected from the underlying pectoralis major muscle. On the lateral chest wall, the long thoracic and thoracodorsal nerves can be seen.

border of the pectoralis minor muscle are carefully identified and preserved. In doing so the medial border of the pectoralis minor is identified. To gain access to the axillary tissue, the fascia along the lateral edge of the pectoralis minor is incised, and the medial pectoral nerve/vessel bundle is isolated, divided, and ligated with 2-0 silk sutures. If only level I and II axillary dissection is to be performed, the pectoralis minor muscle is retracted to expose the apex of level II lymph nodes. Alternatively, if level I to III axillary dissection is to be performed, the pectoralis minor tendon has to be divided to improve exposure. This must be done with care by placing the surgeon's finger beneath the muscle to protect the axillary vessels.

The axillary vein is identified, the adventitial lining over the anterior surface is incised, and the tributaries entering the vein are ligated as they are encountered. If a complete level I to III axillary dissection is to be performed, medial dissection of the axillary vein is extended to its entrance in the thoracic cavity or Halsted ligament. Dissection proceeds laterally until the axillary tissue is freed from the latissimus dorsi tendon. The thoracodorsal nerve, which lies posteromedial to the lateral thoracic vein, is identified and dissected free from the specimen. Along the midaxillary line, the long thoracic nerve of Bell can be seen lying on the chest wall, and it is dissected along its course (see Fig. 11–2). At this point the island of axillary tissue between the two nerves can be grasped and carefully clamped below the axillary vein with two Kelly clamps. The tissue between the two Kelly clamps is divided, and the axillary content is bluntly swept down off the underlying subscapularis.

Finally, the breast tissue is freed from the lateral chest wall. Hemostasis is secured with a combination of electrocautery and 2-0 and 3-0 silk ties. The operative area is thoroughly irrigated with warm saline. Two 10-mm Jackson-Pratt drains are passed through the inferior flap, one placed under the upper flap and the other under the lower flap with its tip in the axilla (Fig. 11–3). The tip must not lie against the axillary vein, because the vein can be damaged by suction.

CLOSURE   The skin flaps are temporarily aligned with the aid of staples. The dermis is approximated with 3-0 absorbable sutures. The skin can then be approximated using subcuticular 4-0 absorbable sutures or staples.

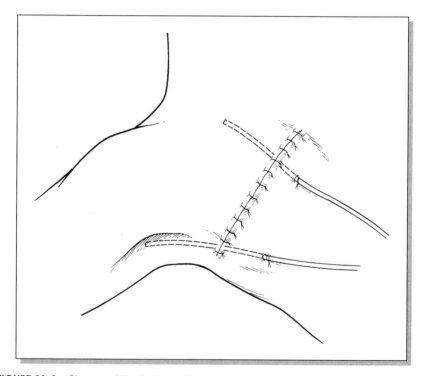

FIGURE 11-3   Closure of the incision after two closed suction drains are placed.

CHAPTER 12

Axillary Lymph Node Dissection

ANATOMY   The axilla is a pyramid-shaped space between the lateral thoracic wall and the upper extremity. Its boundaries are as follows:

Anterior wall: formed superficially by the pectoralis major muscle, and deep to it is the pectoralis minor muscle enclosed by the clavipectoral fascia. The clavipectoral fascia blends with the axillary vessels superiorly.

Posterior wall: composed from above downward by the subscapularis, latissimus dorsi, and teres major muscles.

Lateral wall: the intertubercular groove on the shaft of the humerus to which is attached the pectoralis major, latissimus dorsi, and teres major muscles.

Medial wall: serratus anterior overlying the upper ribs and intercostal spaces.

Base: formed by the skin, subcutaneous tissue, and axillary fascia.

Apex: formed by the outer border of the first rib, superior border of the scapula, and middle third of the clavicle.

Clinically, the axilla is divided into levels using the pectoralis minor muscle as a reference—level I is below, level II is posterior to, and level III is superior to the pectoralis minor muscle (Fig. 12–1). The axilla contains adipose tissue, axillary lymph nodes, the axillary artery/vein

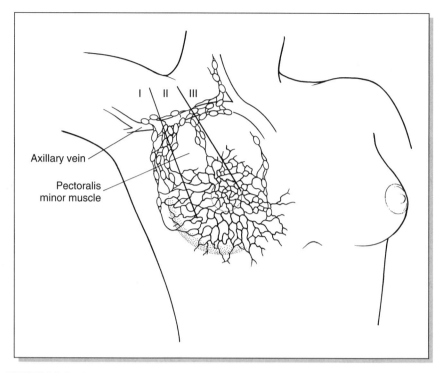

FIGURE 12-1 The levels of axillary lymph node tissue in relation the pectoralis minor muscle.

with the adjacent cords of the brachial plexus, and its terminal branches. Also present are the coracobrachialis and the biceps. The three relevant nerves that travel through the axilla are the long thoracic, thoracodorsal, and intercostobrachial nerves.

The thoracodorsal nerve (C6-8) arises from the posterior cord of the brachial plexus and emerges from beneath the axillary vein to enter the axilla. The nerve travels laterally to meet the subscapular vessels, and in so doing these structures (axillary vein, thoracodorsal nerve, and subscapular vessels) form a triangle over the subscapularis muscle. The thoracodorsal nerve lies superficial to the subscapular artery as it descends along the anteromedial aspect of the latissimus dorsi muscle, which it innervates.

The long thoracic nerve (C5-7) is formed over the first digitation of the serratus anterior muscle and runs vertically downward to enter the axilla. In the proximal part of the axilla, the long thoracic nerve lies superficial to the serratus anterior fascia and is embedded within the fatty tissue. The long thoracic nerve travels medially and approximately at the level of the fourth and fifth intercostal spaces; it pierces this fascia to lie on the surface of the serratus anterior muscle. Along its entire course, the nerve lies behind the midaxillary line, namely posterior to the lateral thoracic perforating vessels.

Operative Procedure

INCISION The lateral border of pectoralis major muscle and the anterior border of latissimus dorsi muscle are palpated and marked with an indelible pen. A skin-crease incision is made just below the axillary hairline and extends from the marked borders of the pectoralis major to the latissimus borders (Fig. 12–2).

EXPOSURE AND OPERATIVE TECHNIQUE The incision is sharply carried through skin and subcutaneous tissue. Using rake retractors to provide traction, the operator creates superior and inferior skin flaps with sharp dissection. Proceeding directly with the main axillary dissection can

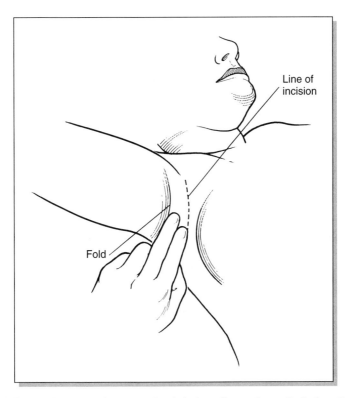

FIGURE 12–2 Incision is made approximately two fingers-breadth below the axillary crease.

prove to be disorienting to an inexperienced operator, and therefore key landmarks need to be identified as the initial step. Richardson retractors are placed at the medial edge of the incision, and the entire length of the lateral border of the pectoralis major muscle is identified. Richardson retractors are placed at the lateral end of the incision, and the antero-lateral border of the latissimus dorsi muscle is identified.

Once the lateral edge of the pectoralis major is dissected free, it is retracted upward with two Richardson retractors. The interpectoral fat, Rotter nodes, and overlying fascia are dissected and included in the speci-men. Next, the fascia at the lateral edge of the pectoralis minor is incised, thus freeing the muscle. The medial pectoral nerve and vessel bundle is isolated, divided, and ligated with 2-0 silk sutures. This maneuver allows the pectoralis minor muscle to be retracted upward to allow access to the axilla. If only levels I and II are to be dissected, adequate exposure can be obtained by retracting the pectoralis minor muscle. Alternatively, if the lymph nodes are grossly positive for metastatic disease, a full axillary dissection (levels I, II, and III) is performed, which requires division of pectoralis minor. To transect this tendon, the index finger is placed behind the pectoralis minor to protect the underlying axillary vein, and the ten-don is divided sharply with electrocautery. Elevation and medial rotation of the arm is helpful in relaxing the pectoralis major muscle and making the axillary dissection easier.

With the pectoralis minor retracted and/or divided, the next step is to identify the axillary vein. Several methods have been described for identi-fying the axillary vein:

- The axillary vein is identified at its highest point, an oval foramen through which the axillary vein enters to become the subclavian vein. This can be felt with the tip of the finger at the medial approximation of the clavicle and the first rib.
- The highest limit of the clavipectoral fascia is palpated, and two fingers-breadth from this point a horizontal incision is made in the fascia. The axillary vein will be seen beneath the upper lip of the divided fascia.
- The white tendon of the latissimus dorsi is followed proximally, and this leads to the axillary vein.
- The costocoracoid ligament (Halsted ligament) is identified, and the clavipectoral fascia is incised inferior to the ligament to reveal the axillary vein.
- The tributaries of the axillary vein can be followed proximally to the axillary vein.

The surgeon should be familiar with all these techniques because they may all prove useful during the axillary dissection. The fascia over the length of the axillary vein is incised. Dissection above the vein must be avoided to preserve the upper extremity lymphatics and prevent the risk of subsequent arm edema. Small venous tributaries entering the axillary vein are ligated with 3-0 silk sutures as they are encountered.

With the pectoralis minor retracted, the lymphatic tissue at level II is carefully dissected off the chest wall. Dissection proceeds by releasing the axillary tissue from the lateral chest wall. The lateral thoracic perforating vessels/nerve bundles that are encountered must be serially divided and ligated with 2-0 silk sutures. The serratus anterior fascia should not be violated because it helps to protect the long thoracic nerve. In fact, at this stage the glistening serratus anterior fascia often becomes folded on the chest wall, and to the untrained eye it can be mistaken for the long thoracic nerve. The search for the long thoracic nerve begins high in the axilla, where it is found embedded within the axillary tissue, lying approximately 1 cm away from the chest wall. The thin layer of adventitial tissue

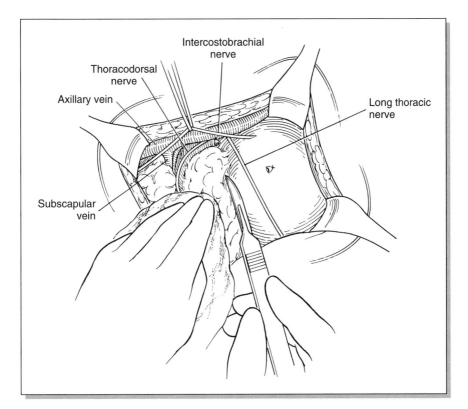

FIGURE 12–3 The important structures exposed during axillary dissection include the axillary vein and the intercostobrachial, thoracodorsal, and long thoracic nerves. With these structures in view, the axillary tissue is dissected off the lateral chest wall.

enveloping the lymphatic tissue is incised lateral and parallel to the long thoracic nerve, thus freeing the nerve, which can then be pushed medially toward the chest wall. The next important step is to identify the thoracodorsal nerve. The lateral thoracic vein, a large venous tributary of the axillary vein, is an important landmark for identification of the thoracodorsal nerve. The thoracodorsal bundle containing the nerve and the vessels is located approximately 1 cm deep and medial to this vein.

At this point, the island of axillary tissue between the two nerves can be grasped and carefully clamped below the axillary vein with two Kelly clamps, keeping the two nerves under constant view (Fig. 12–3). The tissue between the two clamps is divided, and the axillary content is bluntly swept down off the subscapularis muscle. Dissection is continued caudally to remove the axillary content from the groove between the latissimus dorsi muscle and the serratus anterior muscle. The entire axillary content now remains attached at its inferior limit. Therefore, the inferior flap is retracted and the axillary tissue is finally dissected with electrocautery while the two nerves are maintained under view.

CLOSURE   The wound is thoroughly irrigated with warm saline. A 10-mm Jackson-Pratt drain is placed in the axilla through a separate stab incision, ensuring that the tip of the drain is not close to the axillary vein or the nerves. The dermis is approximated with 3-0 absorbable sutures, followed by subcuticular 4-0 absorbable sutures. The closure can be reinforced with Steri-Strips.

Abdomen

ABDOMINAL WALL

CHAPTER 13

Inguinal Hernia Repair

ANATOMY   The inguinal canal is an oblique space measuring 4 cm in length that lies above the medial half of the inguinal ligament. At its medial end there is a triangular opening, called the external inguinal ring, that lies above and lateral to the pubic crest. The internal inguinal ring is located at the lateral end and represents an opening within the transversalis fascia. The boundaries of the internal inguinal ring are superiorly the transverus abdominis arch, inferiorly the iliopubic tract, and medially the inferior epigastric vessels. The thickened fascia overlying the epigastric vessels is called Hesselbach's ligament. The internal inguinal ring is located 1 cm above the femoral artery pulse or midway between the anterior superior iliac spine and pubic tubercle.

The relationships of the inguinal canal are as follows:

Anterior: external oblique fascia along the entire length with contribution from the internal oblique fascia at the lateral one third.

Posterior: fusion of the transversalis fascia and the transversus abdominis fascia.

Inferior (floor): the inguinal ligament and its shelving edge and medially the lacunar ligament of Gimbernat.

Superior (roof): the arch formed by the internal oblique and transversus abdominis muscle (conjoint tendon).

The contents of the inguinal canal include the following:

Male: the spermatic cord travels through the inguinal canal and consists of three nerves, three arteries, and three other structures. The nerves are the ilioinguinal nerve, the genital branch of the genitofemoral nerve, and the sympathetic nerves. The three arteries are the spermatic artery from the aorta, the artery to the vas deferens from the superior vesicle, and the cremasteric artery from the deep epigastric artery. The remaining other three structures include the vas deferens, the pampiniform venous plexus, and the lymphatic channels. The cord has three coverings—the outer external spermatic fascia, the middle cremasteric muscle layer, and the inner internal spermatic fascia—which are derived from the external oblique fascia, internal oblique muscle, and transversus fascia, respectively.

Female: the round ligament of the uterus, ilioinguinal nerve, and genital branch of the genitofemoral nerve.

Several named condensations of fascia or ligaments in relation to the inguinal canal are used during various repairs of inguinal hernias:

Inguinal ligament (Poupart's ligament): This is the condensed lower portion of the external oblique fascia and extends from the anterior superior iliac spine to the pubic tubercle. Its medial third has a free edge, whereas the lateral two thirds are attached to the iliopsoas fascia.

Pectineal ligament (Cooper's ligament): This is a strong ligament attached to the pubic ramus and formed jointly from the aponeurosis of the internal oblique, transversus abdominis, and pectineus muscles.

Iliopubic tract (Thompson's ligament): This is the condensed part of the transversalis fascia and extends from the pectineal ligament medially, forms the inferior border of the internal ring and the anterior wall of the femoral sheath, and attaches laterally to the iliopectineal arch (medial thickening of iliopsoas fascia).

PREOPERATIVE WORK-UP Exacerbating factors contributing to the development of hernia must be identified. These include chronic constipation, chronic cough, prostatic hypertrophy, and any other condition that would chronically elevate intra-abdominal pressure. Appropriate measures must be taken to correct or at least improve these exacerbating conditions preoperatively. This is particularly important in order to achieve lower hernia recurrence rates. A very large inguinoscrotal hernia that contains a large proportion of the intra-abdominal contents is known as loss of domain. Acutely reducing these contents within the abdomen during the process of hernia repair may cause diaphragmatic compromise, leading to postoperative respiratory failure. To prevent this complication, repeated abdominal pneumoperitoneum needs to be undertaken to increase the capacity of the intra-abdominal cavity. In patients with uncontrolled ascites secondary to cirrhosis, elective repair of the hernia may be hazardous because it can lead to hepatic decompensation and death. Before repair of a symptomatic hernia in these patients, placement of a temporary peritoneovenous shunt (LaVeen or Denver shunt) or transjugular intrahepatic portosystemic shunt should be considered.

Patients presenting acutely with a strangulated hernia require emergent operative intervention and therefore are rapidly assessed and resuscitated. Symptomatic incarcerated hernias must be repaired urgently.

In the presence of a large inguinal or inguinoscrotal hernia, it is wise to place a Foley catheter, because the bladder can often become part of the wall of the sliding hernia. Prophylactic antibiotics are administered.

Operative Procedure

POSITION   The patient is placed in the supine position.

ANESTHESIA   For a routine uncomplicated hernia repair, local anesthesia with sedation is generally adequate. In the presence of strangulation or incarceration, general anesthesia is preferred. Alternatively, spinal anesthesia can be used, particularly in elderly patients with comorbid conditions.

INCISION   An incision is usually made parallel to and approximately 2 cm above the inguinal ligament. For adequate exposure the incision should extend from the level of the pubic tubercle to the internal ring at the level of the femoral pulse. Some surgeons prefer a skin-crease incision, which tends to be placed farther away from the pubic tubercle medially and has the disadvantage of causing difficult access to the external ring.

EXPOSURE AND OPERATIVE TECHNIQUE   Numerous methods of hernia repair have been described in the literature: Bassini, McVay, Shouldice, and the tension-free Lichtenstein, to name a few. Interested readers can obtain details in well-known textbooks dealing with the subject. The initial dissection is identical for all procedures, but procedures differ in how the floor of the hernia is repaired.

Before the hernia repair is begun, local anesthesia is administered. Either 1% lidocaine or a mixture containing 1% lidocaine, 0.25% Marcaine, and bicarbonate solution can be used. First the ilioinguinal nerve is infiltrated. This is located approximately 1 cm medial and inferior to the anterior superior iliac spine. Intradermal and the subcutaneous tissues are infiltrated at the site of the proposed incision. The skin and the subcutaneous tissue are incised with a no. 10 scalpel. Two branches of the superficial epigastric veins are invariably encountered; they are clamped, divided, and ligated with 3-0 silk sutures. A self-retaining Weitlaner retractor is placed. At the lateral end of the incision the subcutaneous tissue is further incised until the external oblique fascia is identified. At this point further local anesthesia is infiltrated beneath the external oblique fascia. The rest of the subcutaneous tissue is now incised down to the level of the external oblique fascia. The self-retaining retractor is repositioned.

At this point the external ring is identified on the medial aspect. With a no. 15 scalpel an incision is made into the external oblique fascia along its fibers. The edges of this incision are grasped with Kelly clamps, and the external oblique fascia is carefully dissected free from the underlying areolar tissue and both the ilioinguinal and genitofemoral nerves. While these two nerves are protected, the inguinal canal is opened by extending the incision toward the external ring. The two nerves are then carefully freed, preserved, and retracted out of the way. If needed, these nerves can be directly infiltrated to provide local anesthesia.

The entire cord needs to be carefully freed from the floor of the inguinal canal. This is best started at the level of the pubic tubercle. The operator grasps the cord structures with the left hand, and using the right index finger palpates the pubic tubercle and gently elevates the cord using a combination of blunt and sharp dissection. A quarter-inch Penrose drain is placed around the cord to facilitate retraction. The cremasteric muscles are divided, and the cremasteric artery is ligated to carefully delineate the internal ring. Particular care is taken to avoid injuring the inferior epigastric vessels that are present on the medial border of the internal ring.

To identify the indirect sac, dissection is commenced on the anterolateral aspect of the cord. First, the spermatic coverings arising from the internal oblique and the transversus muscle are divided. A shiny white sac is identified, grasped with hemostats, and dissected free from the cord structures. If the distal end of the sac is visualized, this is also grasped so that the entire sac can be resected. The sac is dissected proximally toward the internal ring. The sac needs to be opened to inspect its contents and to exclude the presence of a sliding hernia (Fig. 13–1). If the distal end of the sac is not visualized, it can be transected at any convenient location along the spermatic cord. The distal end is left open to allow drainage. If the sac is devoid of any abdominal contents, it is twisted and suture ligated at the level of the internal ring with 2-0 absorbable sutures. If, on the other hand, a sliding hernia is present, the sac is trimmed to the level of the sliding structure and closed with continuous 2-0 absorbable sutures.

After the indirect sac has been resected, the internal ring is evaluated. If it is widened due to the presence of the hernia sac and its contents, it

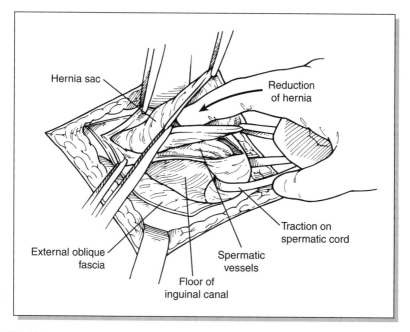

Hernia sac

Reduction
of hernia

Traction on
spermatic cord

External oblique
fascia

Spermatic
vessels

Floor of
inguinal canal

FIGURE 13–1 The hernia sac is dissected free from the cord and then opened to reduce its contents. A Penrose drain placed around the cord provides traction that facilitates dissection.

can be reconstructed with continuous or interrupted 3-0 polypropylene sutures. Once the internal ring is refashioned, it should barely admit the tip of the surgeon's index finger. The internal ring repair should not be made too tight because this can compromise testicular blood supply.

Attention is now directed toward repairing the floor of the inguinal canal. Several methods are described in the literature, as indicated earlier. Some of these repairs are described here.

Bassini Repair The conjoined tendon is retracted upward, and the aponeurosis of the transversus abdominis muscle is approximated to the iliopubic tract that lies adjacent to the inguinal ligament with several interrupted 3-0 silk sutures. The second layer of the repair involves suturing the conjoined tendon to the inguinal ligament with interrupted 2-0 silk sutures. This suture line extends from the pubic tubercle to the medial border of the internal ring. If during this layer of repair a great deal of tension is noted, several small relaxing incisions can be made in the anterior rectus sheath. Several sutures can be used to approximate the conjoined tendon to the inguinal ligament proximal to the cord. However, care must be taken to not constrict the cord.

McVay Repair This is the technique used commonly when there is a large direct inguinal hernia. The attenuated posterior inguinal wall that consists only of thin transversalis fascia is excised, revealing the underlying preperitoneal connective tissue. The segment of posterior wall that is attached to Cooper's ligament should also be excised even though it may appear to be strong. The defect after excision of all the attenuated layers should reveal the preperitoneal connective tissue, Cooper's ligament, pectineus muscle fascia, external iliac and inferior epigastric vessels, and femoral sheath. To allow for tension-free reconstruction of the posterior inguinal wall, a 6- to 7-cm relaxing incision is made in the anterior rectus sheath. There are numerous eponyms associated with this relaxing incision, which brings the transversalis fascia down to Cooper's ligament for suturing and reconstructing the inguinal canal.

Starting at the pubic tubercle, the strong edge of the transverse abdominis aponeurosis is sutured to Cooper's ligament with interrupted 3-0 polypropylene sutures until the femoral vein is reached. The next suture placed is referred to as the transition suture because the transversus abdominis aponeurosis is now sutured to the anterior femoral sheath rather than to Cooper's ligament. From this transition suture the transversalis fascia is approximated to the anterior femoral sheath to the level of the internal ring. The rectus abdominis prevents development of a hernia at the defect in the anterior rectus sheath created by the relaxing incision. The cord is replaced within the inguinal canal.

Shouldice Repair With a no. 15 scalpel an incision is made in the transversalis fascia until the preperitoneal fat can be seen. This incision is extended from the internal ring to the pubic tubercle. The resulting upper transversalis fascia flap is bluntly separated from the underlying pre-peritoneal fat until the thickened edge of the rectus sheath on the deep aspect is visualized and grasped with several Allis clamps. The repair involves placing four lines of sutures. The first suture line is started at the pubic tubercle using 3-0 continuous polypropylene, and the white line is approximated to the free edge of the inferior transversalis fascial flap. At the internal ring the suture is tied and then continued medially by approximating the free edge of the superior flap to the shelving edge of the inguinal ligament. When the pubic tubercle is reached, the suture is tied and divided. The third suture line is started at the level of the internal ring where the conjoined tendon is approximated to the inguinal ligament and tied when the pubic tubercle is reached. Using the same suture, the fourth suture line attaches these same structures to one another and is tied at the level of the internal ring. The cord is replaced within the inguinal canal, and the external inguinal aponeurosis is reapproximated with continuous 2-0 absorbable sutures. The subcutaneous tissue is closed with interrupted 3-0 absorbable sutures. The skin is approximated with subcuticular 4-0 absorbable sutures.

Lichtenstein Tension-Free Mesh Repair If there are any discrete defects within the transversalis fascia, the herniating sac is inverted and the edges of the defect are approximated with interrupted 3-0 polypropylene sutures. For a tension-free mesh repair, the length and width of the floor of the inguinal canal are measured. The polypropylene (Marlex) mesh is fashioned to the shape of the floor of the inguinal canal. An opening is fashioned on the lateral aspect of the polypropylene mesh to allow it to pass around the cord structure at the level of the internal ring. The polypropylene mesh is secured to the floor with continuous 3-0 polypropylene monofilament sutures starting at the pubic tubercle. The retracted ilioinguinal nerves are placed over the mesh. The wound is irrigated and hemostasis achieved, particularly of the cord structure. At this point the patient, if awake, can be asked to cough to test the integrity of the repair.

CLOSURE   The external oblique fascia is reapproximated starting at the external ring using 2-0 absorbable sutures. The subcutaneous tissue is irrigated, and any debris is removed. The skin is approximated with subcuticular 4-0 absorbable sutures, and the testis is gently drawn into the scrotum to avoid iatrogenic undescended testis.

CHAPTER 14

Femoral Hernia Repair

ANATOMY   Relevant to this area is the femoral sheath, a funnel-shaped channel that is formed anteromedially by the continuation of the transversalis fascia, posteriorly by the fascia overlying the psoas and pectineus muscles, and laterally by the iliacus fascia. In the thigh, the femoral sheath fuses with the adventitia of the femoral vessels about 3 cm below the inguinal ligament. The sheath is divided into three compartments by the septa: (1) the lateral compartment, occupied by the femoral artery; (2) the intermediate compartment, occupied by the femoral vein; and (3) the medial compartment, called the femoral canal, which is empty and through which femoral hernia may pass. The femoral canal is about 1 to 2 cm long and communicates superiorly with the retroperitoneal space by an opening referred to as the femoral ring.

The boundaries of the femoral canal (Fig. 14–1A) are as follows:

Anterior: inguinal ligament (Poupart's ligament).

Posterior: pectineal ligament (Cooper's ligament).

Lateral: femoral vein.

Medial: edge of the lacunar (Gimbernat's) ligament. In about 10% of cases, the abnormal obturator artery passes adjacent to the lacunar ligament and may be injured during division of the lacunar ligament.

The femoral canal normally contains fat and a lymph node called Cloquet's node.

PREOPERATIVE PREPARATION Preoperative preparation will depend on the mode of presentation, in particular whether the femoral hernia is incarcerated or strangulated. If the patient has an associated small bowel obstruction, appropriate measures such as placement of nasogastric tube for decompression, intravenous fluid resuscitation, and placement of Foley catheter need to be instituted.

Operative Procedure

POSITION The patient is placed in the supine position. The inguinal area and lower abdomen are prepped and draped in the usual fashion.

EXPOSURE AND OPERATIVE TECHNIQUE The approach for repair of the femoral hernia depends on the mode of presentation.

Low Approach For uncomplicated elective repair of a femoral hernia, the low approach is commonly used. An oblique incision is made over the hernia, approximately one finger-breadth below the medial half of the inguinal ligament (Fig. 14–1B). The incision is carried through the subcutaneous tissue until the hernia sac is encountered. The sac is gently grasped with a Babcock clamp and dissected sharply down to the level of the neck (Fig. 14–2A). At the level of the hernia sac, the femoral vein laterally and the greater saphenous vein entering the femoral vein from its medial side are identified and preserved. The sac is opened and the contents reduced. The neck of the sac is transfixed with 2-0 absorbable sutures with particular care taken to ensure that structures such as bowel and bladder that may form part of the wall are not injured. The femoral canal is repaired with three or four interrupted 2-0 polypropylene monofilament sutures to approximate the inguinal ligament to the pectineal ligament (Fig. 14–2B). Injury to the femoral vein is avoided by retracting this vessel with the index finger while the sutures are placed. Avoid narrowing the femoral vein. An alternative method of repair involves placing into the femoral canal a Marlex mesh plug that is then secured in place with 2-0 polypropylene monofilament sutures.

High Approach (Pre-peritoneal) This approach is preferred if the femoral hernia is strangulated or there is associated small bowel obstruction. An incision can be made in the inguinal region (see Fig. 14–1B). Alternatively, an oblique incision is made along the lateral border of the rectus sheath. The anterior rectus sheath is opened and the rectus muscle is retracted medially. The transversalis fascia is incised and the peritoneum is dissected toward the femoral canal. While counter-pressure is provided in the groin, an attempt is made to gently reduce the hernia sac. If there is still difficulty in reducing the hernia, the medial edge of the femoral ring can be sharply divided. The area must be

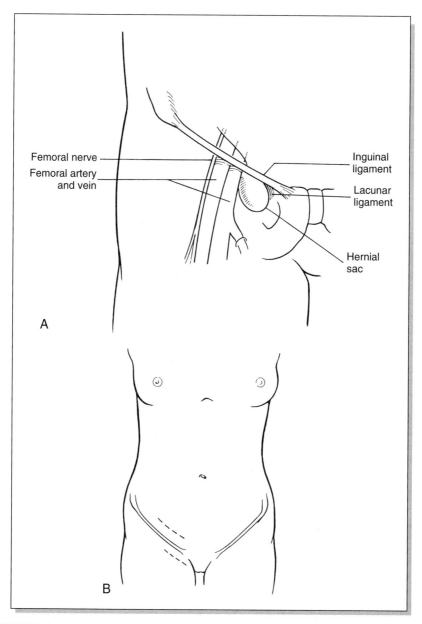

FIGURE 14–1 *A,* Anatomy of the femoral canal. *B,* Incisions used for repair of femoral hernia.

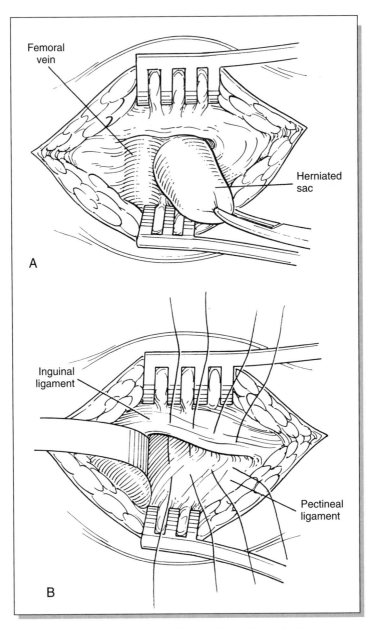

FIGURE 14-2 *A,* The sac is grasped and dissected free; the operator must be cognizant of the femoral vein present on the lateral aspect. *B,* The inguinal ligament is sutured to the pectineal ligament.

inspected for an aberrant obturator artery before the medial edge is incised. The sac is opened and the small intestine is inspected for viability. The compromised bowel is resected if it is nonviable (see Chapter 33). The sac is excised, and the peritoneal defect is closed with 2-0 absorbable sutures. The femoral canal is closed by suturing of the inguinal ligament to Cooper's ligament with 2-0 nonabsorbable monofilament sutures (see Fig. 14–2*B*).

CLOSURE   The anterior rectus sheath is closed with 2-0 nylon sutures. The skin is approximated with staples.

CHAPTER 15

Umbilical/Periumbilical Hernia Repair

EMBRYOLOGY   The umbilicus is the site where the rapidly growing midgut loop extrudes into the extraembryonic coelom in the umbilical cord at the end of the sixth week of development. This represents a temporary "physiologic" hernia, with the loop remaining here for a full month.

ANATOMY   The umbilicus is the site of attachment of the umbilical cord in the fetus. In adults it consists of the umbilical ring that is situated in the linea alba and covered by the umbilical fascia, which represents a thickening of the transversalis fascia. The umbilicus possesses the following important embryologic remains:

1. Median umbilical ligament, the fibrous remnant of the urachus that, if continued patent, would lead to drainage of urine from the umbilicus.
2. Falciform ligament, which contains the ligamentum teres, which is the remains of the obliterated umbilical vein.
3. Persistent vitellointestinal duct leading to a colocutaneous fistula or a fibrous band, which can lead to bowel obstruction.

PREOPERATIVE PREPARATION   Usually minimal preoperative work-up is required unless the patient has ascites secondary to underlying cirrhosis. In these patients avoid repair unless a complication such as rupture with leakage of ascitic fluid or strangulation has occurred.

Operative Procedure

ANESTHESIA Most of these procedures can be performed with local anesthesia and sedation.

POSITION The patient lies in the supine position, and the abdomen is prepped and draped in a sterile fashion.

INCISION For small hernias an infraumbilical curved incision is made (Fig. 15–1A). Alternatively, if the hernia is large with redundant skin, an elliptic incision that removes the umbilicus can be used.

EXPOSURE AND OPERATIVE TECHNIQUE The skin is incised with a scalpel down to the subcutaneous tissue. The hernia sac is identified, and dissection proceeds toward outlining its neck at the level of the fascia. The edge of the defect in the fascia is clearly delineated. The sac is carefully opened and the contents inspected (Fig. 15–1B). In most cases, pre-peritoneal fat can be either reduced or resected. The pre-peritoneal fat is resected if it appears nonviable. The sac is excised to the level of the fascia. The fascial surface is dissected for a distance of at least 1 or 2 cm to allow repair to be conducted safely. The edges of the fascia are grasped with Allis clamps. A standard Mayo-type repair is performed that involves overlapping the superior fold of the fascia on top of the inferior flap in a "double-breasted suit" style using 1-0 polypropylene sutures. If the fascia appears attenuated, consider reinforcing the repair with Marlex mesh. In the presence of ascites, an airtight closure of the fascia is required.

CLOSURE The wound is irrigated, and the dermis is approximated with 3-0 absorbable sutures. The skin is closed with 4-0 subcuticular absorbable sutures.

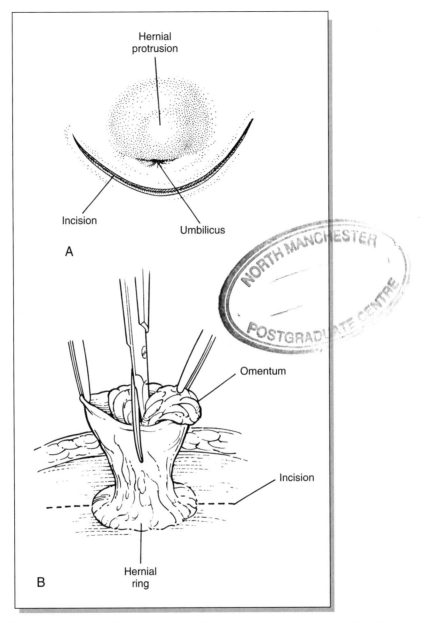

FIGURE 15–1 *A,* A periumbilical incision is made. *B,* The hernia sac is dissected down to the level of the fascia. The content of the sac is inspected.

ESOPHAGUS/STOMACH/
DUODENUM/SMALL BOWEL

CHAPTER 16

Transabdominal Nissen Fundoplication

EMBRYOLOGY AND ANATOMY   See Chapter 19.

PREOPERATIVE PREPARATION   Before the decision is made to perform an antireflux procedure, the presence of gastro-esophageal reflux with all accompanying complications such as reflux esophagitis or stricture formation must be confirmed. The preoperative barium swallow must be reviewed for the presence of a shortened esophagus, esophageal stricture, or abnormal gastric emptying. 24-hour pH monitoring is useful in correlating the patient's pain with episodes of gastric reflux. Because the patient may have been on prolonged H_2 receptor antagonists or proton pump inhibitors, gastric achlorhydria may allow bacterial overgrowth, and thus peri-operative antibiotics should be administered.

Operative Procedure

POSITION   The patient is placed in a supine position and undergoes general anesthesia with endotracheal intubation. The anesthesiologist should be requested to place a nasogastric tube. A Foley catheter is also inserted, and sequential compression devices are placed over the lower extremities.

INCISION   A midline incision from the xiphoid process extending 2 to 3 cm distal to the umbilicus is made.

EXPOSURE AND OPERATIVE TECHNIQUE   Initially, a thorough exploration is performed to exclude any coincident pathology. The stomach and the duodenum are meticulously evaluated for the presence of active ulceration or scars from healed ulcers. The gallbladder is palpated for presence of cholelithiasis.

The patient is placed in the reverse Trendelenburg position, and an upper hand retractor system is arranged to allow the costal margins to be elevated. In addition, a Balfour abdominal wall retractor is placed to provide exposure. If the left lobe of the liver is enlarged or extends far to the left side, the left triangular ligament is divided sharply with electrocautery. The left lobe can thus be folded and retracted away from the esophageal hiatus. The peritoneal covering over the esophageal hiatus is identified and grasped with a long Schnidt clamp. This peritoneal reflection is incised transversely and extended to the left across the whole gastrophrenic ligament and to the right as far as the gastrohepatic ligament. The vagal trunk and branches are identified and preserved. The esophagus is dissected free from its surrounding areolar tissue for a length of approximately 6 cm using a combination of blunt digital dissection and electrocautery. A large Penrose drain is passed around the esophagus to provide traction. If feasible, the posterior vagus trunk should be separated from the esophagus and thus excluded from the fundal wrap. The Penrose drain is retracted downward to determine if adequate gastric fundus is available for the wrap. If the fundus is believed to be inadequate for the wrap, the first two or three short gastric vessels are clamped, divided, and ligated with 2-0 silk sutures. The anesthesiologist is asked to withdraw the nasogastric tube and replace it with a 40 Fr Maloney esophageal dilator.

First, the esophageal hiatus is inspected; if this is believed to be enlarged, the two diaphragmatic crura are approximated with interrupted 2-0 silk sutures. At completion of repair of the esophageal hiatus, it should allow easy passage of one finger through it. With the right hand, the gastric fundus is passed behind the esophagus and grasped with two long Babcock clamps (Fig. 16–1A). Before commencing the wrap, the operator removes the Penrose drain. The fundal wrap should measure approximately 3 to 4 cm in length. The wrap is begun by placing 2-0 silk interrupted seromuscular sutures that include seromuscular bites of the two fundal folds and the esophagus. About four of these sutures are placed at approximately 1-cm intervals and tied down snugly (Fig. 16–1B). To create a floppy Nissen fundoplication, two fingers should easily pass between the wrap and the esophagus. To stabilize the fundal sleeve, two more sutures should be placed at the bottom edge of the fundal wrap and the anterior wall of the stomach.

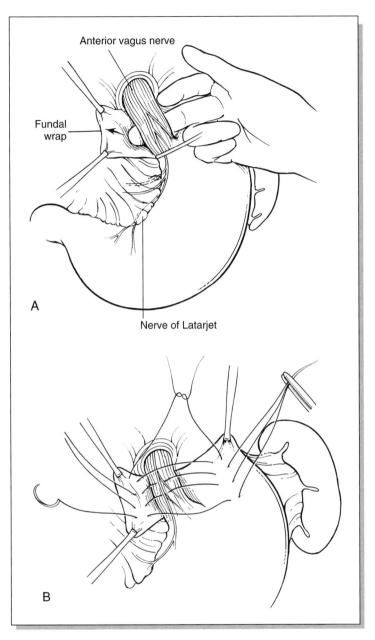

FIGURE 16–1 *A,* The mobilized gastric fundus is passed behind the distal esophagus. *B,* The fundal wrap is constructed by placing at least four sutures, taking bites of the two fundal folds and the esophagus.

The large gastric Maloney tube is removed and replaced with a standard nasogastric tube. The operative region is inspected for hemostasis and for evidence of any inadvertent traumatic injury. The previously ligated short gastric vessels stumps are inspected to ensure that they are well secured. Note that if the patient had been diagnosed as having both gastroesophageal reflux and a gastroduodenal ulcer, Nissen fundoplication can be combined with a highly selective vagotomy, with the vagotomy performed first. The technical description of highly selective vagotomy is described in Chapter 18. The abdominal cavity is irrigated and the position of the nasogastric tube confirmed.

CLOSURE The midline incision is closed in a standard fashion by approximating the linea alba with continuous 1-0 polypropylene monofilament sutures. The skin is approximated with staples.

CHAPTER 17

Laparoscopic Nissen Fundoplication

EMBRYOLOGY AND ANATOMY　See Chapter 19.

Operative Procedure

PREOPERATIVE PREPARATION　This is the same as an open Nissen fundoplication (see Chapter 16).

POSITION　The patient is placed in the lithotomy position to allow the surgeon to operate between the legs of the patient. This allows comfortable access to the esophageal hiatus.

INCISION AND ESTABLISHMENT OF PNEUMOPERITONEUM　A transverse skin-crease incision is made above the umbilicus, and blunt dissection of the subcutaneous tissue is performed to identify the linea alba. Using two towel clips, the operator grasps the skin and abdominal wall and inserts a Veres needle through the fascia into the peritoneal cavity. The tip of the Veres needle should be directed toward the feet of the patient to avoid inadvertent injury to the abdominal aorta. To confirm presence of the needle within the abdominal cavity, a drop test is performed: while the abdominal wall is pulled up with the towel clamps, a drop of saline is placed in the hub of the needle. The drop of saline should fall rapidly if the tip of the Veres needle is within the peritoneal cavity. Intra-abdominal insufflation is initiated, and the initial pressure reading should remain relatively low. High pressures early during insufflation indicate that the needle probably is improperly placed and should be repositioned or reinserted. If there is still concern regarding the position of the Veres needle, the surgeon should resort to an open technique using the Hassan cannula. In the open technique, after two stay sutures are placed using 0-0 absorbable sutures, the linea alba is incised and the peritoneal cavity entered. Under direct vision, the Hassan cannula with the blunt-tipped trocar is placed. If, however, insufflation is progressing well, the abdominal cavity should rise and be uniformly tympanitic on percussion. The intra-abdominal pressure should be observed to rise gradually. Once the intra-abdominal pressure has reached about 15 mm Hg and approximately 2.5 to 3 L of CO_2 has been insufflated, the Veres needle is removed.

PLACEMENTS OF PORTS Four operating ports are placed along a semicircle opposite the xiphoid process. The assistant on the right side of the patient operates the camera. The patient is placed in a steep reverse Trendelenburg position.

EXPOSURE AND OPERATIVE TECHNIQUE After placement of all ports, an opening is made into the gastrohepatic ligament and extended over the intra-abdominal esophagus. The dissection around the esophageal hiatus is similar to that for the open procedure. The two crura are clearly identified, and the lower 3 to 4 cm of the abdominal esophagus is mobilized. The esophagus is retracted to the right, and the crural defect is closed with interrupted silk sutures. To avoid excessive tightness of the crural closure, a 60 Fr Maloney bougie is placed in the esophagus.

Next, with the aid of a harmonic scalpel, the fundus and the proximal aspect of the greater curvature are freed by dividing the short gastric vessels (Fig. 17–1). A Penrose drain is placed around the abdominal esophagus to elevate it toward the anterior abdominal wall. This opens the retroesophageal space, through which the assistant can grasp the previously freed fundus and pass it beneath and to the left side of the esophagus. Finally, the fundal wrap, measuring approximately 2 cm, is sutured in a similar manner to that described for the open technique.

Once the procedure is completed, the area of the esophageal hiatus is irrigated with saline. The port sites are removed under direct vision.

CLOSURE The fascial defects at the periumbilical and infraxiphoid locations are closed with figure-of-eight sutures using 0-0 absorbable sutures. The skin is approximated with subcuticular 4-0 absorbable sutures and reinforced with Steri-Strips.

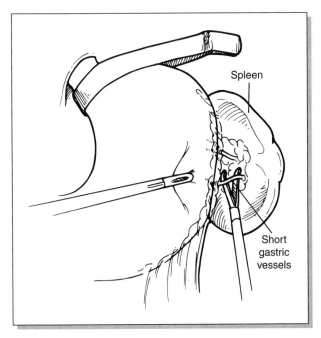

FIGURE 17-1 The stomach is grasped to provide traction while the short gastric vessels are divided commonly with a harmonic scalpel. A Penrose drain is placed around the abdominal esophagus.

CHAPTER 18

Vagotomy and Drainage Procedures

EMBRYOLOGY AND ANATOMY　See Chapter 19.

Operative Procedure

Truncal Vagotomy and Drainage

POSITION　The patient is placed in the supine position and undergoes general anesthesia with endotracheal intubation. A nasogastric tube and a Foley catheter are placed.

INCISION　A midline upper abdominal incision is preferred because it allows good access to the esophageal hiatus (Fig. 18–1).

EXPOSURE AND OPERATIVE TECHNIQUE　A thorough exploration is first performed to evaluate for evidence of chronic inflammation of the stomach or duodenum. The gallbladder is evaluated for evidence of chronic cholecystitis or cholelithiasis. Once the exploration is complete, an upper hand retractor is used to elevate the costal margins. To improve access to the esophageal hiatus, the left triangular ligament is sharply divided with electrocautery, and the left lateral lobe of the liver is carefully retracted or folded. A transverse incision is made in the peritoneum overlying the esophagus at the hiatus in the diaphragm. This opening is then widened on each side of the esophagus by

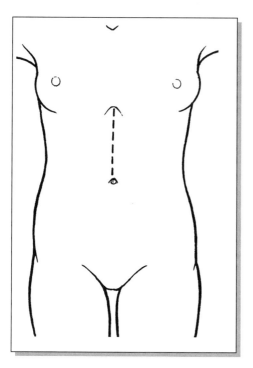

FIGURE 18–1 Midline incision used for performing vagotomy and drainage procedures.

sharply dividing the adjacent lesser omentum and the esophagophrenic ligament. Blunt dissection is continued until two or three fingers can be comfortably passed around the esophagus (Fig. 18–2).

Using a large right-angle Mixter clamp, a one-half-inch Penrose is passed around the esophagus. The anterior (left) vagal trunk is then sought and may be palpated. It can also be seen as a taut yellow cord lying on the anterior surface of the esophagus (see Fig. 18–2). Downward traction on the stomach and esophagus with the aid of the Penrose renders this vagal trunk more prominent.

The anterior trunk is separated from the esophagus with the aid of a right-angle Mixter clamp or a nerve hook. Two hemoclips are placed along the anterior vagal trunk, and a segment of the nerve between the clips is excised and sent to the pathologist for frozen section. With the right hand behind the esophagus, the operator locates the posterior (right) vagal trunk (see Fig. 18–2, *inset*). The posterior vagus is usually felt as a stout cord lying behind and to the right of the esophagus. The nerve is carefully freed, again two hemoclips are placed on the nerve trunk to isolate a segment, and approximately 1 cm of the nerve is excised and sent for frozen section examination (see Fig. 18–2, *inset*). After transecting the vagal trunks, it is essential to clear the distal 5 to 6 cm of the esophagus by meticulously dissecting and dividing all strands of nerve

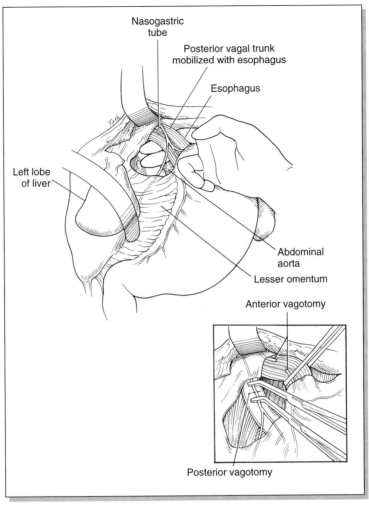

FIGURE 18–2 The left lobe of the liver is retracted to expose the esophageal hiatus. The distal esophagus is mobilized at the hiatus to reveal the anterior vagal trunk. Two fingers are passed behind the esophagus to locate the posterior vagal trunk. *Inset,* The posterior vagal trunk is divided.

fibers, small blood vessels, and fascia. The criminal nerve of Grassi, which is a branch of the posterior vagus to the fundus, must be sought diligently and divided in the usual fashion. After completion of this extensive periesophageal dissection, only the longitudinal esophageal fibers should be visible. Such meticulous dissection is essential to ensure complete vagotomy and subsequent low incidence of recurrent ulceration. If a selective vagotomy is to be performed, the hepatic branch of the anterior vagus nerve and the celiac division of the posterior vagus nerve are preserved.

The esophagus is retracted to the left and the diaphragmatic hiatus assessed. If the hiatus allows more than two fingers, it is repaired with interrupted 2-0 silk sutures. At completion of the hiatal dissection, a moist laparotomy pad is placed for hemostasis and attention is directed toward performing the drainage procedure.

The type of drainage procedure performed depends on the condition of the duodenum. Usually a pyloroplasty is considered standard practice, but if the duodenum is scarred and inflamed, a gastrojejunostomy is a suitable alternative.

Pyloroplasty

When undertaking a pyloroplasty, a Kocher maneuver is first performed to mobilize the second part of the duodenum. Two 2-0 silk stay sutures are placed at the superior and inferior aspects of the pylorus. A 6- to 10-cm transverse incision is made starting from the antrum and extending across the pylorus and into the first part of the duodenum. This incision is closed longitudinally with an inner layer of interrupted 3-0 absorbable sutures encompassing all layers, followed by a seromuscular layer of 3-0 silk Lembert sutures. Alternatively, a stapled closure can be performed. In this case, the edges of the incision are grasped in a longitudinal fashion with several Allis clamps. The incision is closed with a TA-55 stapler containing 4.8-mm staples.

Gastrojejunostomy

To construct a gastrojejunostomy, first a loop of jejunum approximately 12 to 15 cm from the ligament of Treitz is selected and brought through an opening in the transverse mesocolon usually to the left of the middle colic vessels. The stoma should be placed in the prepyloric region or at the most dependent portion of stomach. Using 3-0 silk, a posterior layer of seromuscular Lembert sutures is placed. Before opening the bowel, non-crushing Doyen clamps are placed on both sides of the proposed anastomosis to occlude the jejunum. The area of the anastomosis is isolated with moist laparotomy pads in case there is spillage of jejunal contents. In addition, the suction catheter must be readily available to contain any possible spillage. The stomach and the adjacent jejunum are opened. Using 3-0 absorbable sutures, the full-thickness inner layer is started posteriorly and completed anteriorly using inverting Connell sutures. Placing an anterior seromuscular layer of interrupted 3-0 silk Lembert sutures completes the anastomosis.

For a stapled anastomosis, the jejunum is first aligned to the dependent portion of the stomach with 2-0 silk stay sutures at each end. A stab incision is made in the stomach and jejunum, and the anastomosis is performed using a GIA-60 stapling device. The staple line is inspected for hemostasis. The combined stab incision is closed with an inner layer of continuous 3-0 absorbable sutures and an outer layer of interrupted 3-0 silk Lembert sutures. Finally, the transverse mesocolon is carefully closed around the anastomosis to avoid herniation.

Billroth I and II Gastrectomy

If an antrectomy is to be performed as part of the antiulcer procedure, dissection is commenced along the distal half of the greater curvature. First, the greater omentum is separated from the proximal half of the transverse colon. The greater omentum is carefully separated from the transverse mesocolon to avoid any traction injury to the middle colic vessels during subsequent dissection. Next, the branches from the gastroepiploic arcade to the greater curvature are divided and ligated with 2-0 silk sutures from the midportion of the stomach to the duodenum. As this dissection proceeds toward the duodenum, the small fragile vessels are ligated in continuity with 3-0 silk sutures and divided. Meticulous dissection in this region will avoid any unnecessary bleeding or injury to the pancreas.

With gentle dissection using a Schnidt clamp, the posterior wall of the first part of the duodenum is freed from the pancreas and divided with a GIA-60 linear stapler. The right gastric artery is identified above the pylorus, divided, and ligated with 2-0 silk sutures. With electrocautery the gastrohepatic ligament is divided proximally along the lesser curvature. Just proximal to the incisura angularis, the left gastric vessels lying along the lesser curvature are carefully isolated with a right-angle Mixter clamp. These vessels are individually ligated in continuity with 2-0 silk sutures and divided. Proximally these vessels are suture ligated with 3-0 silk sutures. After the nasogastric tube is withdrawn proximally, the stomach is divided with a GIA-90 linear stapler.

If adequate length of supple duodenum is available, a Billroth I gastroduodenal anastomosis can be constructed (Fig. 18–3). The staple line along the transected duodenum is sharply excised and hemostasis is controlled. A two-layer anastomosis, with an outer layer of interrupted Lembert 3-0 silk sutures and an inner layer of full-thickness continuous 3-0 absorbable sutures, is performed. The gastric staple line from the lesser curvature is inverted with 3-0 silk interrupted Lembert sutures until the "angle of sorrow" of the gastroduodenal anastomosis is reached, where a crown suture is placed.

If a Billroth II gastrojejunostomy (Polya-Hoffmeister type) is to be constructed, a loop of proximal jejunum is selected and brought in an antecolic or retrocolic fashion toward the transected stomach. The loop of jejunum is aligned along the lower half of the gastric staple line with 3-0 silk stay sutures. For a hand-sewn anastomosis, first a posterior layer of interrupted 3-0 silk Lembert sutures is placed, approximating the posterior

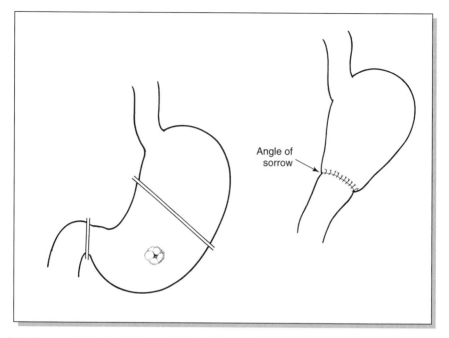

FIGURE 18–3 Antrectomy followed by Billroth I gastroduodenostomy has been performed. The "angle of sorrow" where anastomotic leak can occur is shown.

wall of the stomach and the jejunum. Noncrushing bowel clamps are placed on the small bowel. With electrocautery a longitudinal enterotomy is made in the loop of jejunum, and the appropriate length of adjacent gastric staple line is sharply excised. An inner layer of continuous 3-0 absorbable sutures is placed. Finally, the anterior interrupted Lembert 3-0 silk sutures are placed to complete the anastomosis.

Next, the gastric staple line from the lesser curvature is inverted with 3-0 silk interrupted Lembert sutures until the angle of sorrow of the gastrojejunal anastomosis is reached, where a corner crown suture is placed. For additional security at this location, the adjacent jejunal wall can be used to cover the angle of sorrow (Fig. 18–4). For a stapled Billroth II anastomosis, stay sutures are placed to hold the loop of jejunum adjacent to the gastric remnant. A small stab incision is made in the jejunum and at the adjacent posterior wall along the greater curvature of the stomach. The limbs of the GIA stapler are inserted and fired. It is important to have at least 2 cm of posterior gastric wall between the gastric staple line and the gastrojejunostomy to avoid necrosis.

The anastomosis is inspected for any bleeding. Finally, the stab wound is approximated with a series of Allis clamps, ensuring that any existing staple lines are staggered. The defect is closed with a TA-55 stapler. The staple line can be inverted with interrupted Lembert 3-0 silk sutures.

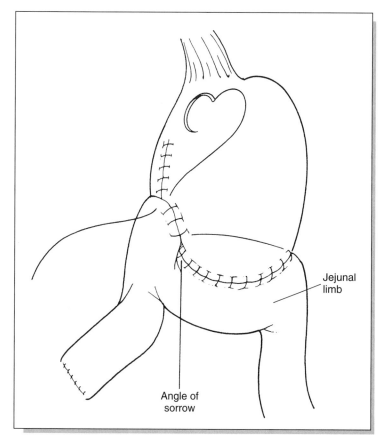

FIGURE 18–4 Billroth II gastrojejunostomy after either a distal or subtotal gastrectomy.

CLOSURE The midline abdominal incision is closed in the standard fashion as described before.

Highly Selective Vagotomy

The position, incision, and initial exploration are as described for truncal vagotomy and pyloroplasty. First, the anterior nerve of Latarjet is identified, which can be seen leaving the gastroesophageal junction and running downward in the lesser omentum parallel to the lesser curvature and terminating at the incisura angularis (5–7 cm from the pylorus) as several branches resembling a crow's foot. These terminal branches and the branches from the nerve of Latarjet to the body of the stomach are accompanied by the blood vessels. The posterior vagal trunk also runs downward within the lesser omentum as the posterior nerve of Latarjet, and its course and distribution to the posterior aspect of the stomach are similar to those of the anterior nerve of Latarjet.

Before the anterior dissection is begun, the lesser sac needs to be inspected for any adhesions to the pancreas that could be inadvertently avulsed during dissection, leading to bleeding. To enter the lesser sac, the gastrocolic ligament is sharply divided but the gastroepiploic arcade is kept intact. Any avascular congenital adhesions present between the stomach and the pancreas are divided with electrocautery. A nasogastric tube is placed by the anesthesiologist and should be directed toward the antrum, so it can be used to grasp the greater curvature and provide downward traction.

The dissection commences at the site just proximal to the crow's foot on the anterior aspect of the stomach. The objective is to divide the lesser omentum from the lesser curvature, between the incisura angularis and the esophagus, by dividing all the blood vessels and the accompanying nerves that enter the lesser curvature. The anterior layer of the lesser omentum, adjacent to the neurovascular bundle, is sharply incised. With the use of a fine Schnidt clamp, the neurovascular branches are carefully dissected, ligated in continuity with 3-0 or 4-0 silk sutures, and divided. This dissection proceeds proximally up along the lesser curvature until the left side of the gastroesophageal junction is reached.

Next, the stomach is turned upward, and again the nasogastric tube is used to grasp the greater curvature. The posterior denervation is conducted in a similar fashion. Attention is then turned to performing a careful and meticulous dissection of the lower 5 cm of the esophagus, which is conducted by ligating and dividing all blood vessels and nerve fibers entering the esophagus, particularly on its right lateral and posterior aspects. By dividing close to the wall of the upper stomach and lower esophagus, damage to the main vagal trunk and its celiac and hepatic branches is avoided.

The two critical components of achieving a successful and a complete highly selective vagotomy are (1) separation of the lesser curvature of the stomach completely from the lesser omentum, extending from the incisura angularis to the cardia, and (2) skeletonizing the lower 5 to 7 cm of the esophagus.

CLOSURE The midline abdominal incision is closed in the standard fashion described before.

CHAPTER 19

Gastrectomy

EMBRYOLOGY The anatomic relationships of the stomach in the adult can be easily understood by the embryologic development. The stomach is derived from the foregut. It is initially a fusiform dilatation present in the median plane that subsequently undergoes two rotations. A 90-degree rotation occurs along the longitudinal axis of the stomach such that the left side forms the anterior surface, and the right side the posterior surface. The original ventral border forms the lesser curvature, and the faster growing dorsal border develops into the greater curvature. This rotation results in the left vagus' innervating the anterior surface and the right vagus' innervating the posterior surface of the stomach. A further rotation occurs in the anteroposterior axis, allowing the stomach to assume the transverse position in relation to the long axis of the body. The primitive lesser sac (omental bursa) is derived from resorption of the right side of the thick dorsal mesogastrium. The lesser sac is located behind the stomach in adults, and this position results from expansion of the bursa, lengthening of the dorsal mesogastrium, and rotation of the stomach. The lesser sac communicates with the general peritoneal cavity through the epiploic foramen (foramen of Winslow).

ANATOMY The stomach is the dilated portion of the foregut between the esophagus and the duodenum. It is usually J shaped and located in the left upper quadrant and epigastrium, and its distal part can extend to the level of the umbilicus. The stomach is divided into a fundus, body, antrum, and pylorus. The fundus is that part of the stomach that lies above the level of the gastroesophageal junction. The body extends from the fundus to the incisura angularis. The incisura angularis is most clearly seen during gastroscopy. The pyloric portion of the stomach consists of the antrum, which extends from the incisura angularis to the proximal limit of the pylorus. The pyloric canal is surrounded by a thick muscular wall that forms the pyloric sphincter. The pyloric canal is approximately 2.5 cm long, and the pyloroduodenal junction is identified by presence of the prepyloric vein (vein of Mayo), which crosses its anterior surface.

The stomach possesses a lesser and a greater curvature. The lesser curvature extends from the right side of the esophagus to the level of the pylorus, and to it is attached the lesser omentum (gastrohepatic ligament). Conversely, the greater curvature extends from the left of the esophagus, around the fundus, and to the right side of the pylorus. The upper part of the greater curvature gives attachment to the gastrosplenic ligament containing the short gastric vessels, whereas the greater omentum extends from the lower portion of the greater curvature. The posterior relation of the stomach, also known as the bed of the stomach, is formed by the lesser sac. Posteriorly, the relations are the diaphragm above and, from right to left, the pancreas, the splenic artery, the spleen, the left kidney, and the adjacent adrenal gland.

Because the stomach is derived from the foregut, its blood supply originates from the branches of the foregut artery, the celiac axis. The left gastric artery that arises from the celiac axis and the right gastric artery that arises from the hepatic artery supply the lesser curvature and the adjacent surfaces. The greater curvature and the adjacent portion of the stomach are supplied by the left gastroepiploic artery, which arises from the splenic artery, and from the right gastroepiploic artery, which arises from the gastroduodenal branch of the hepatic artery. The short gastric arteries arise from the splenic artery at the hilum, pass within the gastrosplenic ligament, and supply the fundus. The venous drainage of the stomach flows through the portal vein. The right and the left gastric veins enter the portal vein directly, the right gastroepiploic vein drains into the superior mesenteric vein, and the left gastroepiploic vein and the short gastric veins join the splenic vein. The lymphatic drainage follows the arteries and drains ultimately into the celiac lymph nodes.

The nerve supply of the stomach is derived from both the right and the left vagus nerve and the celiac plexus of sympathetic fibers that arise from the fifth, sixth, seventh, and eighth thoracic segments of the spinal cord. Because of the rotation of the stomach during embryonic development, the left vagus lies anterior to the esophagus, whereas the right vagus lies posterior. The anterior vagus enters the abdomen anterior to the esophagus and gives off hepatic branches that travel in the lesser omentum to supply the liver and the gallbladder and a branch through the pyloric antrum. The anterior vagus nerve continues along the lesser omentum as the nerve of Latarjet and terminates approximately 5 to 7 cm proximal to the pylorus in several branches, described as the crow's foot. The posterior (right) vagus nerve also lies between the leaves of the lesser omentum and follows a course along the lesser curvature posterior to the anterior vagus nerve as the nerve of Latarjet. In 90% of the cases, the posterior vagus nerve gives rise to the nerve of Grassi, which originates at the level of the gastroesophageal junction and supplies the gastric fundus.

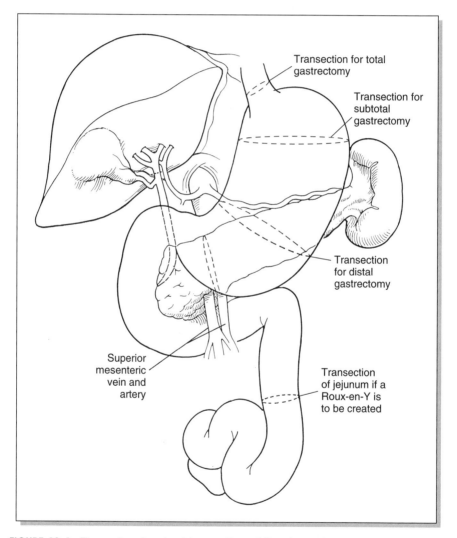

FIGURE 19–1 The various levels of transection of the stomach needed to perform a total, subtotal, or distal gastrectomy. The level of jejunal transection needed to construct a Roux-en-Y jejunal limb is shown.

However, in up to 20% of cases, the nerve of Grassi may actually originate above the hiatus. When performing truncal vagotomy it is important to identify and divide this branch to minimize the incidence of recurrent ulceration.

A total, subtotal, or distal gastrectomy is performed, depending on the location of the tumor and whether an adequate en bloc lymphadenectomy can be performed (Fig. 19–1).

PREOPERATIVE PREPARATION Tissue diagnosis must be obtained, and the extent of the malignant disease, particularly extension in the esophagus, is determined with preoperative upper gastrointestinal endoscopy. Basic laboratory tests are obtained. Computed tomography of the abdomen, pelvis, and chest is performed to completely stage the disease. If there is cardiac history, a preoperative stress echo or Persantine thallium scan is obtained to assess the ejection fraction and cardiac wall motion. For a proximal tumor with extension into the esophagus, the thoracic cavity may need to be accessed; therefore, pulmonary function tests are obtained. If a computed tomography scan of the abdomen suggests extension of the disease to the transverse colon, a mechanical bowel preparation is performed, because bowel resection may be necessary.

RADICAL TOTAL GASTRECTOMY

This procedure is most commonly performed for malignant diseases of the stomach.

Operative Procedure

POSITION The patient is placed in the supine position. If there is likelihood of performing a thoracoabdominal incision, the patient's left side is elevated with a wedge. A nasogastric tube and Foley catheter are inserted, and preoperative prophylactic antibiotics are administered.

INCISION Adequate exposure can be obtained with a long midline incision. If necessary, an oblique extension into the left chest wall can be performed to improve exposure of the distal esophagus in the left thoracic cavity.

EXPOSURE AND OPERATIVE TECHNIQUE After entering the abdominal cavity, the operator's first step involves assessing whether the disease is curable surgically by evaluating the presence of liver metastasis, peritoneal implants (particularly those that are outside the confines of the resection such as in the pelvis and diaphragm), and para-aortic lymph nodes. In the presence of incurable disease, palliative gastrectomy should be considered if the patient is symptomatic from the tumor.

The mobility of the spleen is assessed because subsequent medial displacement of the organ facilitates dissection of the short gastric vessels. Any obvious adhesions are carefully divided to prevent traction injury to the splenic capsule. The greater omentum is lifted and separated from the transverse colon along the avascular plane and carefully dissected free from the transverse mesocolon up to the level of the pancreas. As the greater omentum is retracted superiorly, the right gastroepiploic branch of the gastroduodenal artery and the accompanying vein are encountered adjacent to the head of the pancreas. These vessels are carefully dissected, divided, and ligated. The perigastric tissue in the region of the pylorus is dissected superiorly to include the subpyloric nodes within the specimen. Multiple small vessels are encountered adjacent to the duodenum. These vessels are serially clamped with fine hemostats, divided, and ligated with 3-0 silk sutures. The proximal greater curvature of the stomach is mobilized by dividing the left gastroepiploic artery. To facilitate the dissections of the short gastric vessels, the gastrosplenic ligament can be brought into view by displacing the spleen medially and packing the splenic bed with moist lap pads. This has the added benefit of avoiding traction on the spleen, thus avoiding inadvertent injury. The short gastric vessels are individually isolated, clamped, and ligated with 2-0 silk sutures. On the gastric side the vessels are further secured with 3-0 silk transfixion suture ligatures.

Attention is now directed toward mobilizing the esophagus. First, the left triangular ligament of the liver is divided with electrocautery, thus allowing the left lateral lobe to be retracted. This maneuver exposes the esophageal hiatus. The peritoneal reflection over the hiatus is opened to expose the two diaphragmatic crura. With careful blunt digital dissection, the esophagus is encircled and a Penrose drain is placed for traction. The left hand is passed behind the esophagus and the esophagophrenic ligament is divided, thus completing the mobilization of the fundus and greater curvature of the stomach. The distal esophagus within the posterior mediastinum is carefully mobilized. The two vagi are identified and divided between hemoclips. The lesser omentum is divided to expose the celiac axis and its major branches. The left gastric artery is identified near its origin and divided after ensuring that the left hepatic artery does not originate from the left gastric artery. The peritoneum over the porta hepatis is dissected to identify the right gastric artery, which is clamped, divided, and ligated. After the duodenum is mobilized with a Kocher maneuver, the first part of the duodenum is dissected from the head of the pancreas and transected with the GIA-60 linear stapler. This allows the stomach to be elevated and any posterior congenital adhesions to be divided.

Normally it is not necessary to resect the spleen during the total gastrectomy unless bulky lymph nodes are encountered in the splenic hilum, in which case the spleen is removed en bloc. If the spleen is to be removed, it is drawn medially, and the splenocolic, splenorenal, and phrenosplenic ligaments are divided sharply with electrocautery. This has the added benefit of allowing assessment of the tail of the pancreas. If the tail of the pancreas is grossly involved with tumor, it is mobilized by dissecting in the retropancreatic space and is transected proximal to the area of involvement with the use of a TA-55 stapler. At this point the specimen should be left attached solely at the esophageal end. A right-angle bowel clamp is placed over the distal esophagus. Two stay sutures are placed in the esophageal wall just proximal to the clamp using 0-0 silk. The esophagus is divided, and the specimen is sent to the pathologist to perform frozen section analysis of both the distal and proximal margins.

Lymphadenectomy is performed by skeletonizing the celiac, splenic, and hepatic arteries. About 15 to 20 cm from the duodenojejunal flexure, the jejunum is divided with a GIA-60 linear stapler. The mesentery is divided to allow the distal aspect of jejunum to reach the esophagus without tension. If further length of jejunum is required, the peritoneal lining of the mesentery is incised in several directions. A 2- to 4-cm opening is made in the avascular segment of the transverse mesocolon, and the distal jejunal loop is passed through the defect toward the esophagus. The esophagojejunal anastomosis can be either hand sewn or constructed with the EEA stapling device.

For a hand-sewn end-to-side anastomosis, the outer posterior layer of interrupted Lembert sutures using 3-0 silk is placed between the esophagus and the jejunum. The adjacent antimesenteric border of the jejunum is opened with electrocautery. An inner full-thickness layer of interrupted 3-0 silk sutures is placed. Finally, the outer anterior layer of interrupted seromuscular Lembert sutures using 2-0 silk is placed to complete the anastomosis.

If a stapled anastomosis is being constructed, the transected esophagus is gently dilated either digitally or with the 25 Fr sizer provided with the stapling device. A purse-string suture is placed around the esophagus using a 3-0 polypropylene monofilament suture. The anvil of the EEA stapler is placed in the esophagus, and the purse-string suture is tied down snugly. Next, the staple line at the end of the distal jejunal limb is excised to allow insertion of the EEA stapler. The EEA stapling instrument is opened to advance the central rod through an antimesenteric stab wound located approximately 3 to 4 cm from the end of the jejunal limb (Fig. 19–2A). The anvil is engaged to the central rod; the EEA is closed and then fired. The EEA is again opened and gently removed. The two tissue doughnuts are inspected to ensure that they are complete. The anastomosis is inspected for hemostasis, and the jejunum is closed with a TA-55

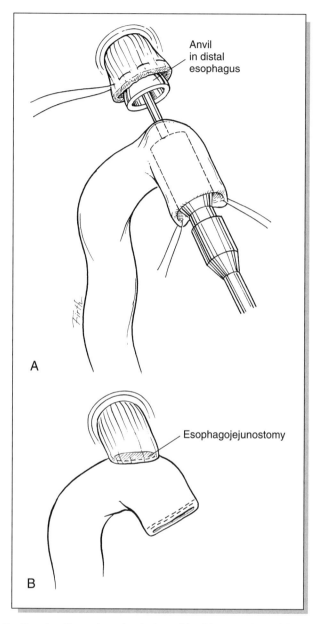

FIGURE 19–2 Construction of a stapled end-to-side esophagojejunal anastomosis. *A,* The anvil is passed into the esophagus and the purse-string suture is tied. *B,* The completed end-to-side esophagojejunal anastomosis.

stapler (Fig. 19–2*B*). The anastomosis is tested by having the anesthesiologist inject methylene blue through the nasogastric tube while gently occluding the small bowel. The areas of leaks are reinforced with interrupted 3-0 silk sutures. The anastomosis is secured anteriorly with a second layer of seromuscular suture using 3-0 silk sutures. The nasogastric tube is passed beyond the anastomosis.

A side-to-side jejunojejunostomy is constructed approximately 50 cm distal to the esophagojejunostomy. To prevent internal herniation, defects in the transverse mesocolon are closed. At a convenient place distal to this jejunojejunostomy, a feeding jejunostomy catheter is placed. A drain is placed in the region of the transected duodenum and close to the pancreas if it has been transected.

CLOSURE The midline incision is closed in a standard fashion by approximating the linea alba with continuous 1-0 polypropylene monofilament sutures. The skin is approximated with staples after the subcutaneous tissue has been irrigated and hemostasis achieved.

RADICAL SUBTOTAL GASTRECTOMY

For small cancers limited to the distal antrum, the patient can be offered radical distal or subtotal gastrectomy. At initial exploration, determination of resectability is similar to that described for total gastrectomy.

Operative Procedure

EXPOSURE AND OPERATIVE TECHNIQUE The omentum is separated from the transverse colon along the avascular plane and carefully lifted from the transverse mesocolon to the level of the pancreas. The right gastroepiploic branch of the gastroduodenal artery and the right gastroepiploic vein are encountered adjacent to the head of the pancreas. These are carefully isolated, divided, and ligated. The perigastric tissue that contains the subpyloric nodes in the region of the pylorus is included with the specimen. Multiple small vessels encountered adjacent to the duodenum are clamped with fine hemostats, divided, and ligated with 3-0 silk sutures. The first part of duodenum is carefully freed and then transected with a linear GIA-60 stapler. The gastrohepatic ligament is incised close to the liver to be included with the specimen. For a distal gastrectomy, at least a 5-cm proximal margin from the tumor is achieved. However, if the tumor extends into the body of the stomach or up the lesser curvature, a total gastrectomy is needed.

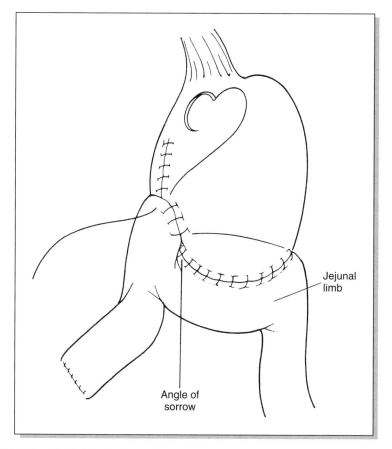

FIGURE 19–3 Billroth II gastrojejunostomy after either a distal or subtotal gastrectomy.

After the site of transection of the stomach is determined, the descending branch of the left gastric vessels along the lesser curvature and the left gastroepiploic vessels along the greater curvature are carefully isolated, ligated in continuity with 2-0 silk, and divided. The stomach is transected with either a GIA-90 linear or a TA-90 stapler. The specimen is sent to pathology for frozen section analysis of the proximal and distal margins. Once margins have been determined to be clear of tumor, a standard Billroth II gastrojejunostomy is constructed as outlined for benign condition (Fig. 19–3), except that it should be antecolic.

CLOSURE The midline incision is closed in a standard fashion by approximating the linea alba with continuous 1-0 polypropylene monofilament sutures. The skin is approximated with staples after the subcutaneous tissue has been irrigated and hemostasis achieved.

CHAPTER 20

Gastrostomy

EMBRYOLOGY AND ANATOMY   See Chapter 19.

Operative Procedure

INCISION   Usually, a gastrostomy is placed as part of another intra-abdominal procedure. Currently, most gastrostomies are performed using the percutaneous endoscopic technique.

Stamm Gastrostomy

EXPOSURE AND OPERATIVE TECHNIQUE   The body of the stomach is grasped with two Babcock clamps. An inner purse-string suture of 2-0 absorbable suture is placed, followed by an outer purse-string suture using 2-0 silk (Fig. 20–1A and B). The adjacent linea alba is grasped with Kocher clamps, and with a no. 10 scalpel a skin stab incision is made in the region of the rectus sheath. A long Schnidt clamp is passed through this stab incision into the peritoneal cavity under direct vision. Using this Schnidt clamp as a guide, a similar clamp is passed from the peritoneum outward through the same incision. An 18 Fr Foley catheter or a gastrostomy tube is drawn through the anterior abdominal wall using the Schnidt clamp. With electrocautery, a gastrotomy is made in middle of the previously placed inner purse-string suture, and the tip of the Foley catheter is inserted into the stomach. The balloon is inflated with 10 to 20 mL of water, and the purse-string sutures are snugly tied down.

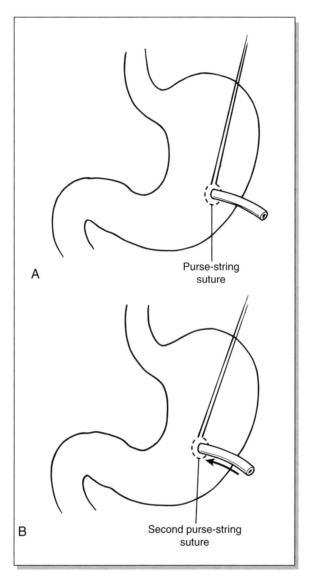

FIGURE 20–1 *A,* The inner purse-string suture is tied down after the gastrostomy tube is passed into the stomach. *B,* The second, outer purse-string suture is tied.

The gastrostomy tube is secured to the anterior abdominal wall at four quadrants with the 2-0 silk suture (Fig. 20–1*C*). The gastrostomy tube is flushed with saline. The tube can be secured to the skin with a 3-0 nylon suture.

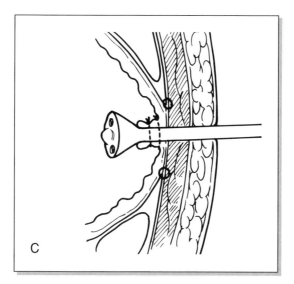

FIGURE 20–1 *Continued.* C, Cross-section shows the gastrostomy tube being brought out through the anterior abdominal wall, and the anterior stomach wall is sutured to the peritoneum.

Janeway Gastrostomy

This procedure involves creation of a small, permanent gastric tube using the anterior wall of the stomach.

EXPOSURE AND OPERATIVE TECHNIQUE The midportion of the anterior wall of the stomach is grasped with two Babcock clamps and drawn upward. A GIA-60 linear stapler is applied to the serosal surface of the stomach with the tips of the forks about 3 cm from the greater curvature. The instrument is closed and fired, creating an approximately 4- to 5-cm gastric tube. For additional security, the staple line is inverted with interrupted 3-0 silk sutures, taking care to avoid narrowing the lumen of the tube. The gastric tube is brought out through a stab wound in the anterior abdominal wall. The gastric tube is secured on the undersurface of the anterior abdominal wall at four corners using 2-0 silk sutures. The tip of the gastric tube is transected and then matured by placing interrupted mucocutaneous 3-0 absorbable sutures. The gastric tube can be tested by gently passing a Foley catheter through it.

CLOSURE The midline incision is closed in the standard fashion by approximating the linea alba with continuous 1-0 polypropylene monofilament sutures. The subcutaneous tissue is irrigated, and the skin is approximated with staples.

CHAPTER 21

Perforated Peptic Ulcer

PREOPERATIVE PREPARATION   The diagnosis of perforated peptic ulcer is most often evident from the history and physical examination. The accompanying finding of free air on an upright chest radiograph or decubitus abdominal film also supports the diagnosis. The stomach is emptied via nasogastric tube, and a Foley catheter is placed to monitor fluid resuscitation. Intravenous infusion of fluids is begun, and broad-spectrum antibiotics are administered. In select cases, insertion of a central venous line or a Swan-Ganz artery catheter may be necessary for accurate fluid resuscitation and monitoring. As soon as the patient has been adequately resuscitated, emergent exploratory laparotomy should be performed.

Operative Procedure

POSITION   The patient is placed in the supine position, and general anesthesia with endotracheal intubation is instituted.

INCISION   An upper midline incision extending from the xiphoid to just below the umbilicus provides the most expeditious entry into the abdominal cavity. The incision can be extended to the symphysis pubis if necessary.

EXPOSURE AND OPERATIVE TECHNIQUE   Once the abdomen is entered, the free gastric and bilious material is cultured and then evacuated. A careful examination of the stomach and the duodenum is performed to determine the site of perforation. If the anterior surface of the stomach and duodenum does not show any abnormality, the gastrocolic ligament is serially divided between clamps to allow entrance into the lesser sac and inspection of the posterior surface of the stomach. The operative procedure performed depends on variables such as presence of shock, life-threatening comorbid conditions, the degree of contamination of the upper abdomen, the amount and duration of perforation, and whether there is a history or intraoperative evidence of chronic peptic ulceration.

In the presence of life-threatening comorbid conditions and severe intra-abdominal contamination, the safest technique for an acute anterior duodenal perforation is a simple closure with a Graham patch using omentum. Several full-thickness simple sutures are placed across the perforation using 2-0 or 3-0 silk sutures (Fig. 21–1A). A segment of omentum that will easily reach the area of the perforation is placed over the perforation (Fig. 21–1B). The silk sutures are secured. To prevent omental necrosis, the knots should not be tightly secured; however, if the sutures are tied down too loosely, the omentum may slip out, leaving the perforation uncovered. If there is minimal contamination of the upper abdomen and the patient is stable, a definitive ulcer procedure can be performed. For a perforated duodenal ulcer this may include a highly selective vagotomy, a truncal vagotomy and pyloroplasty, or vagotomy and antrectomy (see Chapter 18 for a description of these procedures). Finally, the abdomen is irrigated with a copious amount of warm saline, particularly above the liver.

For a perforated gastric ulcer, the procedure performed will again depend on the condition of the patient. If the patient is moribund, the ulcer is best excised by grasping it with multiple Allis clamps and using a GIA-60 linear stapler. Alternatively, the ulcer can be excised with electrocautery, and the defect is approximated with a two-layer closure with inner continuous 3-0 absorbable sutures and outer interrupted Lembert sutures using 2-0 or 3-0 silk sutures. In a stable patient the ulcer is excised and sent for frozen section analysis to exclude the presence of malignancy. In the presence of a malignant process, an appropriate oncologic resection is performed. For a benign gastric ulcer, a distal gastrectomy with either a Billroth I gastroduodenostomy or a Billroth II gastroduodenostomy is performed. Alternatively, the ulcer can be excised and a truncal vagotomy and drainage procedure performed (see Chapter 18 for description of these operative procedures).

CLOSURE The midline incision is closed by approximating the linea alba with 1-0 absorbable or nonabsorbable monofilament sutures. If excessive contamination has been present, the wound is left open and the subcutaneous tissue should be packed with saline-soaked sterile gauze. If the wound appears clean, a delayed primary closure can be performed on the fifth postoperative day.

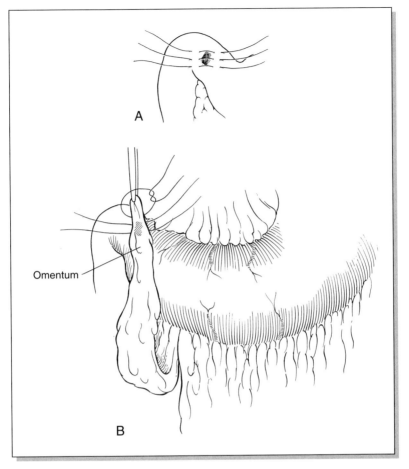

FIGURE 21-1 *A,* Technique of performing a Graham patch. Multiple seromuscular 2-0 or 3-0 silk sutures are placed adjacent to the edges of the perforated ulcer. *B,* A segment of omentum is placed over the perforation, and the sutures are tied down.

CHAPTER 22

Bleeding Duodenal Ulcer

PREOPERATIVE PREPARATION   Patients in whom nonoperative management of a bleeding peptic ulcer has failed will require exploratory laparotomy for hemorrhage control. The patient should be resuscitated with fluids, blood, and blood products. Any associated coagulopathy should be corrected. A nasogastric tube and Foley catheter are placed. Insertion of a central venous line or a Swan-Ganz pulmonary artery catheter is undertaken according to the clinical situation. The site of bleeding may already have been confirmed by endoscopy.

Operative Procedure

POSITION   The patient is placed in the supine position, and general anesthesia with endotracheal intubation is instituted.

INCISION   An upper midline incision is made extending from the xiphoid to below the umbilicus; the incision can be extended to the symphysis pubis as needed.

EXPOSURE AND OPERATIVE TECHNIQUE   Within the abdomen, the stomach is usually found distended with blood, and the small bowel appears a dark blue-gray color due to blood within its lumen. Two stay sutures of 2-0 silk are placed into the duodenum, which is then opened longitudinally, as for a pyloroplasty. The stomach and duodenum are suctioned to identify the site of bleeding. The bleeding site can be manually compressed with gauze to control the bleeding to allow the anesthesiologist to resuscitate the patient as needed.

Control of bleeding from a posterior duodenal ulcer is achieved by suturing the gastroduodenal artery as it passes behind the duodenum. To perform this, a 2-0 silk suture is used on a large, strong, curved needle. A U-shaped suture is placed at the site of the bleeding vessel. Further simple sutures using 2-0 silk are placed above and below the bleeding point (Fig. 22–1). The sutures are firmly secured, making sure that the bleeding has been controlled. Blood clots are emptied from the stomach and duodenum, and a truncal vagotomy and pyloroplasty is performed (as described in Chapter 18). If the patient is hemodynamically stable, after oversewing of the bleeding gastroduodenal vessel a truncal vagotomy and antrectomy is performed because this procedure is associated with the lowest rate of recurrent bleeding (see Chapter 18 for details).

CLOSURE The linea alba is closed with 1-0 monofilament nonabsorbable sutures, and the skin is approximated with staples.

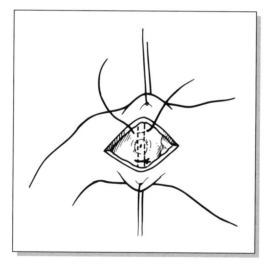

FIGURE 22-1 Hemorrhage from a duodenal ulcer is controlled with sutures placed above and below the bleeding point.

CHAPTER 23

Small Bowel Resection

EMBRYOLOGY   The small intestine arises from the midgut. The midgut begins immediately distal to the origin of the hepatic diverticulum and terminates at the proximal two thirds of the transverse colon. The midgut elongates rapidly to form the primary intestinal loop, with the vitellointestinal duct being present at its apex. The jejunum and the proximal ileum develop from the cephalic limb of the loop, whereas the distal ileum is derived from the caudal limb. The superior mesenteric artery, the artery of the midgut, lies within the longitudinal axis of the intestinal loop. Because the cephalic limb grows relatively rapidly compared with the caudal limb, it causes a 180-degree rotation around the axis formed by the superior mesenteric artery. The jejunum and the ileum continue to elongate and form coiled loops.

As the abdominal cavity becomes too small to contain the midgut, it enters the extraembryonic coelom within the umbilical cord, referred to as the physiologic umbilical herniation. After the expansion of the abdominal cavity and probably reduced growth of the liver, the small bowel reenters the abdominal cavity at the end of the third month. The proximal part of the jejunum is the first segment to reenter the abdominal cavity and comes to lie on the left side. The subsequent parts of the bowel settle more and more to the right side. The mesentery of the jejunum and ileum is at first located in the median plane of the posterior abdominal wall. With elongation, rotation, and reentry into the abdominal cavity, the mesentery becomes fan shaped and the base extends obliquely from the duodenojejunal flexure in the left upper quadrant to the ileocecal area in the right lower quadrant.

ANATOMY   The small bowel extends from the stomach to the colon and consists of the duodenum, jejunum, and ileum. The jejunum and ileum measure approximately 260 cm and extend from the duodenojejunal junction to the ileocolic junction. The upper two fifths are jejunum, and the lower three fifths are ileum. The entire small intestine is covered by visceral peritoneum and is suspended by its mesentery, which extends obliquely from the left side of the second lumbar vertebra to the right sacroiliac joint. Along the oblique course of the root of the mesentery, it crosses the left psoas, aorta, inferior vena cava, right gonadal vessels, right psoas, and right ureter.

The blood supply to the small intestine is derived from branches of the superior mesenteric artery. There is notable difference in the vascular arcades between the jejunum and the ileum. In the jejunum the mesenteric vessels form usually one or two arcades, with long infrequent vessels passing into the intestinal wall. Conversely, the ileum has three or four or more vascular arcades from which numerous shorter terminal vessels arise and supply the bowel wall.

Some other distinguishing features can be used to differentiate between the jejunum and ileum. The jejunum is wider, is thicker walled, possesses larger plicae circularis, and lies in the upper part of the abdominal cavity and to the left side of the transverse mesocolon. By comparison, the ileum has smaller and more widely separated plicae circularis with frequent lymphoid aggregation known as Peyer patches. The ileum lies in the lower half of the abdominal cavity and in the pelvis. There is also a difference in the deposition of the mesenteric fat: in the jejunum it is primarily near the root of the mesentery, and in the ileum the mesenteric fat is deposited throughout so that it extends from the root to the intestinal wall.

The venous drainage of the small intestine corresponds to the arterial supply derived from the superior mesenteric artery and drains into the superior mesenteric vein. The lymphatic drainage includes a large number of mesenteric nodes that finally reach the lymph nodes around the superior mesenteric artery.

Operative Procedure

INCISION   A midline incision provides good exposure and allows extension if any other intra-abdominal bowel pathology is found incidentally.

EXPOSURE AND OPERATIVE TECHNIQUE   A self-retaining Balfour retractor is placed. Next, a thorough exploration is performed, and the entire small bowel from the duodenojejunal flexure to the ileocecal area is carefully inspected. If the small bowel resection is being performed for a malignant tumor, the abdomen is carefully explored for enlarged mesentery lymph nodes and peritoneal implants. The liver is examined for metastatic lesions. The diseased segment of small bowel is identified and elevated out of the abdomen. Moist laparotomy pads are placed to isolate the length of small bowel and also to prevent inadvertent intra-abdominal contamination. Approximately 5 cm of normal bowel on each side of a malignant tumor should be resected. Such wide margins, however, are not required for benign inflammatory processes or traumatic injury, where gross clearance to normal pliable small bowel is adequate.

The site for proximal and distal small bowel transection is selected. From these sites the peritoneal covering on the two sides of the mesentery is incised in a V shape either with electrocautery or with Metzenbaum scissors. By lifting the small bowel, the surgeon may use transillumination to view the vascular arcades. These vessels are carefully dissected, serially clamped, divided, and ligated with 3-0 silk sutures (Fig. 23–1A). For a

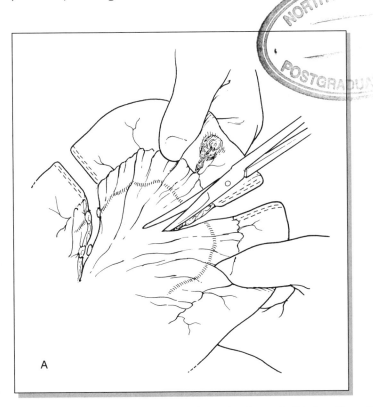

FIGURE 23-1 *A,* The small bowel is divided proximally and distally with a GIA-60 stapler, and the mesenteric vessels are divided and ligated.

Illustration continued on the following page

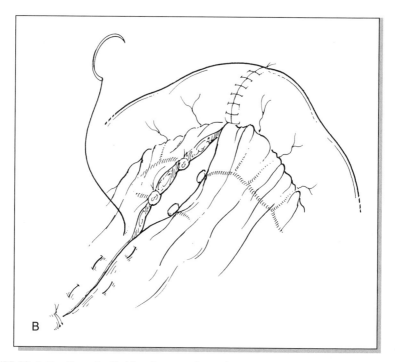

FIGURE 23–1 *Continued.* *B,* After the anastomosis is complete, the mesenteric defect is closed to avoid internal hernia.

faster resection the mesentery can be serially transected with an endovascular linear stapler; alternatively, large hemoclips are placed on the side of the mesentery that will accompany the resected small bowel. In cases in which the mesentery is fatty and edematous, the vessels should be further secured with transfixion suture ligature using 3-0 silk. The small bowel is transected proximally and distally with a GIA-60 stapler (see Fig. 23–1*A*). Next, after gently milking the contents of the small bowel away from the stapled ends, the operator places soft noncrushing Glanzman clamps. The small bowel anastomosis can be either stapled or hand sewn, but it is important to adhere to good surgical principles to allow for healing of the anastomosis. This includes ensuring good blood supply, absence of tension, noncrushed bowel ends, and adequate seromuscular suture placement.

For a two-layer hand-sewn anastomosis, first the posterior layer of interrupted Lembert seromuscular 3-0 silk sutures is placed and the corner stitches are held with hemostats. The staple line is excised with Mayo scissors, and the contents of the small bowel are suctioned. An inner layer of continuous locking hemostatic sutures using 3-0 absorbable material is begun in the back row starting in the center and continued anteriorly with the Connell suture. The anastomosis is completed by placing the anterior seromuscular layer of interrupted Lembert sutures using 3-0 silk.

For a single-layer anastomosis, interrupted 3-0 silk Lembert sutures are placed, starting in the back row and completing the anterior layer in a similar fashion.

To construct a side-to-side stapled anastomosis, the two ends of the small bowel are first aligned by placing 3-0 silk stay sutures. The staple line is excised at the antimesenteric border of the two bowel ends. The limbs of the GIA-60 stapler are passed through the enterotomies, and the stapler is closed and fired. The anastomosis is inspected for hemostasis before closing of the enterotomy with a TA-55 stapler or by hand sewing. The mesenteric defect is closed with continuous or interrupted 3-0 absorbable sutures (Fig. 23–1*B*).

CLOSURE The midline abdominal incision is closed in a standard fashion by approximating the linea alba with continuous 1-0 polypropylene monofilament sutures. The subcutaneous tissue is irrigated with saline, and hemostasis is secured before approximating the skin with the staples.

HEPATOBILIARY SYSTEM

CHAPTER 24

Open Cholecystectomy

EMBRYOLOGY   The liver diverticulum is derived from the distal end of the foregut and grows into the septum transversum. The connection between the hepatic diverticulum and the foregut (which develops into duodenum) elongates and narrows to form the bile ducts. The gallbladder and the cystic duct develop from a ventral outgrowth that emerges from the bile duct. The biliary tree passes through a solid stage that is followed by recanalization. The gallbladder initially is a hollow organ but becomes solid due to proliferation of epithelial cells. Later, recanalization occurs, and failure of this process leads to atresia of the gallbladder.

RELEVANT SURGICAL ANATOMY   The gallbladder is a pear-shaped organ about 7.5 to 10 cm in length. It lies within a fossa on the inferior aspect of the right lobe of the liver. Anatomically it can be divided into a fundus, body, infundibulum, and neck. The fundus extends beyond the edge of the liver and comes in contact with the anterior abdominal wall at the level of the tip of the ninth rib. The infundibulum sags down toward the duodenum at Hartmann's pouch, where gallstones often become impacted. Originating from the neck of the gallbladder is the cystic duct, which joins the common hepatic duct in a variable fashion. The surgically important triangle of Calot is formed by the common hepatic duct on the left, the cystic duct on the right, and the liver above.

The common hepatic duct is formed by the union of the right and the left main bile ducts outside the confines of the liver. It is 2 to 3 cm long and lies entirely within the portal fissure. The common bile duct (CBD) is formed by the union of the common hepatic duct and the cystic duct. It measures approximately 8 cm in length (range, 5–15 cm), and its course is as follows:

- One third in the lesser omentum: It lies anterior to the portal vein with the hepatic artery on the left.
- One third behind the first part of duodenum: It lies anterior to the portal vein, with the gastroduodenal artery on the left.
- One third behind the head of pancreas: It lies over the inferior vena cava.

Behind the head of the pancreas the CBD is joined by the main pancreatic duct to form a common channel known as the ampulla of Vater. The ampulla opens on the posteromedial aspect of the second part of the duodenum. This opening, known as the duodenal papilla, is located approximately 10 cm from the pylorus. This papilla will normally allow passage of a 3-mm dilator. On cholangiography the normal diameter of the CBD ranges from 8 mm to 1 cm, whereas on ultrasonography it is 6 cm.

The blood supply of the gallbladder is derived from the cystic artery, which is most commonly a branch of the right hepatic artery, and lies within the triangle of Calot. The cystic artery tethers the gallbladder and can be felt as a taut string when the gallbladder is retracted laterally. The blood supply of the extrahepatic bile ducts originates from the superior pancreaticoduodenal artery, hepatic artery, and cystic artery. The veins from the gallbladder drain directly into the liver or into the hepatic vein via the pericholedochal plexus.

The foramen of Winslow is an important anatomic landmark for performing the Pringle maneuver. Its relations are as follows: (1) anteriorly, the free border of the lesser omentum; (2) posteriorly, the inferior vena cava and the right adrenal gland; (3) superiorly, the caudate process of the liver; and (4) inferiorly, the horizontal part of the hepatic artery and below it the second part of the duodenum.

PREOPERATIVE PREPARATION Apart from assessment of the cardiopulmonary systems to evaluate the patient's ability to withstand open cholecystectomy, special circumstances should be addressed. If the patient is jaundiced, in addition to the baseline laboratory investigations, liver function tests, hepatitis profile, and a coagulation profile should be obtained. If there is a history of fluctuating jaundice in male patients, Gilbert disease must be excluded. If endoscopic retrograde cholangiopancreatography or percutaneous transhepatic cholangiography has been performed, the results should be reviewed.

Prophylactic antibiotics should be administered, especially for high-risk patients with the following parameters: age older than 70 years and a history of diabetes mellitus, jaundice, CBD stones/stricture, biliary tree malignancy, or steroid usage.

Operative Procedure

POSITION   The patient undergoes general anesthesia with endotracheal intubation. A nasogastric tube is inserted. The patient is placed in a supine position on an x-ray operative table and arranged for ultra-operative fluoroscopy. The patient is prepped and draped. The surgeon should stand on the right side of the table.

INCISIONS   If it is an elective procedure and no other pathology is suspected, it would be appropriate to use a Kocher (oblique right upper quadrant) incision. If on laparotomy other pathology is discovered, a Kocher incision can be extended into a bilateral subcostal incision.

Kocher Incision   A subcostal incision is made. The anterior rectus sheath is incised and the rectus muscle identified. A Rochester-Pean clamp is placed under the muscle, which is divided with electrocautery. The assistant should be ready to clamp epigastric vessels within the rectus muscle, and these vessles are ligated with 2-0 silk sutures. Next, the posterior sheath is incised, and the preperitoneal fat is separated digitally or with hemostats. The peritoneum is grasped with two hemostats and incised to open the peritoneal cavity. The falciform ligament can be spared if the exposure is adequate, but in most cases it is divided and ligated with 2-0 absorbable sutures.

Midline Incision   The linea alba, identifiable by the crisscrossing of the fascial fibers, is incised, and the preperitoneal fat is identified. The peritoneum is grasped up with two hemostats and incised after it has been ensured that no bowel has been inadvertently included with the peritoneal lining. The opening is extended with the use of electrocautery.

EXPOSURE AND OPERATIVE TECHNIQUE   First, a careful exploration is performed to exclude unrecognized pathology, with special reference to "Saint's triad," which is defined by the presence of gallstones, hiatus hernia, and diverticular disease. Other common causes of upper abdominal pain that should be excluded include peptic ulcer, carcinoma of the stomach, carcinoma of the pancreas, and chronic pancreatitis.

Exposure of the gallbladder is achieved through the following steps:

1. Elevate the head of the bed to 15 degrees, which allows the gallbladder to descend into the field of operation.

2. The operator places his or her hand over the liver on the right side to break the suction between the diaphragm and liver, therefore allowing the liver to descend.

3. Using moist laparotomy pads, the operator should (1) pack the hepatic flexure down, (2) pack off the lesser curvature of the stomach to the left, (3) place wet laparotomy pads and use a Deaver or Harrington retractor medial to the gallbladder to retract the liver, and (4) use an additional laparotomy pad to pack off the small intestine and duodenum and have the assistant retract the duodenum.

The above steps are extremely important in facilitating the remainder of the procedure.

Any adhesions present between the gallbladder and the adjacent structures are carefully and sharply divided. The cystic duct and the gallbladder are gently palpated to feel for any stones. The operator should avoid inadvertently dislodging any stones into the CBD. After Hartmann's pouch has been identified, it is grasped with a Rochester-Pean clamp and retracted laterally to place the cystic duct on tension (Fig. 24–1). An additional Rochester-Pean clamp is placed near the fundus to provide traction during dissection. The assistant should retract the duodenum downward

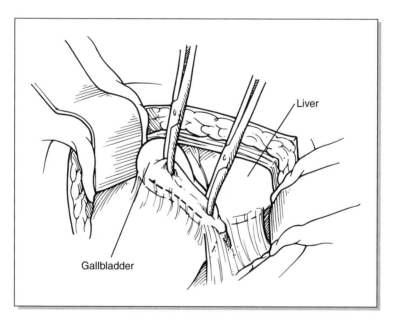

Liver

Gallbladder

FIGURE 24–1 The gallbladder is grasped with two clamps and retracted laterally to expose the triangle of Calot.

to place the CBD on tension. This greatly facilitates the dissection that needs to be performed in Calot's triangle. If there is evidence of intense inflammation or fibrosis in this area, inadvertent injury to the structures within the porta hepatis may occur. In this situation it is wise to first perform the cholecystectomy in the retrograde fashion, where the gallbladder is dissected from its bed, until the cystic duct is clearly identified. Dissection should be undertaken close to the gallbladder wall to avoid injury to the right hepatic artery, right hepatic duct, or CBD.

In the absence of such inflammation, the peritoneal reflection over Calot's triangle is incised gently and reflected toward the liver. The peritoneum is bluntly dissected off the ducts in two opposing directions using a Kittner dissector. It is preferable not to use sharp dissection in this area. By using blunt dissection the cystic duct is identified and the junction between the cystic duct and the CBD is clearly displayed.

Next, the cystic artery is identified and traced down toward the gallbladder. Any vessel that is more than 2 mm in diameter may be the right hepatic artery and therefore should be clearly identified as the cystic artery before division. The cystic artery is dissected free with a right-angle Mixter clamp and doubly ligated with 2-0 absorbable sutures. Alternatively, if the access is difficult, hemoclips can be used. In the event of bleeding from the area of the porta hepatis, avoid blind clamping and instead perform the Pringle maneuver. This maneuver involves passing the forefinger and the middle finger of the left hand through the foramen of Winslow, with the thumb placed anteriorly to compress the hepatic artery within the free edge of the lesser omentum.

Next, an operative cholangiogram is performed. Using a right-angle Mixter clamp, two 2-0 silk ligatures are placed around the cystic duct. The proximal ligature is tied down and held with a hemostat for retraction. One throw of a knot is loosly placed on the distal ligature and held with a hemostat. With Metzenbaum scissors an oblique incision is made in the cystic duct. Patency of the cystic duct is checked with a lacrimal duct probe, which also assists in dilating the valves of Heister, if present. A sample of the bile is sent for culture. A small cholangiocatheter is placed through the aperture while flushing with saline to prevent entry of air bubbles. Now the previously placed distal silk ligature is tied down to secure the catheter. The syringe containing the contrast material is attached to the cholangiocatheter. To prevent entry of air bubbles, the tip of the cholangiocatheter should be below the level of the CBD, and in this position bile should be seen flowing out of the catheter. Next, all the instruments and sponges are removed from the operative field because these can obscure the cholangiogram. With the operating table tilted 10 degrees to the right side, two radiographs are obtained, one after 5 mL and the other after 10 mL of the dye is injected.

The features examined in an operative cholangiogram are

- Normal-caliber CBD (10 mm)
- Free flow into the right and left hepatic ducts
- Absence of any filling defects or strictures
- Narrowing of the distal end of the CBD
- Free flow into the duodenum
- No evidence of leakage from the biliary tree

Once a normal operative cholangiogram is confirmed, then, as described before, the gallbladder and the biliary tree are exposed using moist laparotomy pads and retractors are replaced. A small sponge is placed in the hepatorenal pouch to absorb any blood or bile soiling that may result from the ensuing dissection. The distal ligature is cut using a no. 11 scalpel and the catheter withdrawn. Hemoclips are placed on the cystic duct, and the duct is divided. The preferable length of the cystic duct stump is approximately 0.5 cm.

The gallbladder now remains to be removed in the retrograde fashion. A Schnidt clamp is placed on the cystic duct and retracted laterally. This opens up a plane of dissection between the gallbladder and its bed, which can be further opened with a combination of sharp and blunt digital dissection. The peritoneal covering of the gallbladder and the associated loose areolar tissue are divided with electrocautery. Once the gallbladder is removed, hemostasis is secured with the aid of electrocautery. The gallbladder bed is inspected particularly for any bile leakage from accessory bile ducts of Luschka. If a leak is found, it can be controlled with a figure-of-eight suture using a 3-0 absorbable suture or electrocautery. If there is still some oozing from the gallbladder bed, it is safer to place a hemostatic agent such as Avitene or Surgicel. The operative area is irrigated with saline to remove any debris. If the field is dry and the dissection was easy, there is no need to place a drain. If a drain is placed, its tip is directed into Morison's pouch, because this is the most dependent part of the intra-abdominal cavity where fluid tends to accumulate.

CLOSURE

Kocher Incision The posterior sheath is closed with 1-0 or 2-0 absorbable sutures. The anterior sheath is approximated with a 1-0 nonabsorbable monofilament suture. Skin is closed with staples.

Midline Incision The linea alba is approximated with 1-0 polypropylene or polydioxanone monofilament sutures. Skin is closed with staples.

Exploration of the Common Bile Duct

Initially, the second part of the duodenum is mobilized with a wide Kocher maneuver. The CBD and the common hepatic duct are carefully dissected to allow clear visualization of the biliary system. Below the cystic duct entry, two 4-0 silk stay sutures are placed. An opening in the CBD is made with a no. 11 scalpel, followed by a 1- to 1.5-cm longitudinal incision with Pott scissors. Note that a horizontal incision should not made because such an incision could damage the blood supply to the CBD, which runs along a 3 o'clock and 9 o'clock position.

The CBD is initially flushed with saline solution through a red rubber Robinson catheter distally and proximally. Any stones present within the biliary tree are carefully extracted with the use of Desjardins/Randall forceps. The ducts are flushed with saline solution. Next, the red rubber Robinson catheter is gently advanced through the sphincter and into the duodenum, where the tip can be palpated. If this proves to be difficult, a 14 Fr biliary Fogarty catheter may be used. In addition, 1 mg of glucagon can be administered to relax the sphincter. As the catheter is withdrawn, the ducts are further flushed with saline solution. Some surgeons prefer to use a Bakes dilator, which is gradually passed into the CBD and directed toward the ampulla and into the duodenum.

Finally, the biliary system is inspected with a choledochoscope. If a choledochoscope is not available or if there are concerns during endoscopy, a cholangiogram must be obtained to confirm complete removal of all the biliary calculi. Next, a T-tube is selected according to the diameter of the CBD, which can range from 10 to 14 Fr. The T-tube is prepared by shortening the arms of the T-tubes and excising a wedge opposite the main stem of the tube to facilitate its subsequent removal. The short arms of the T-tube are carefully placed in the CBD and the opening closed with 4-0 absorbable sutures. These sutures are placed above the exit site of the T-tube, because sutures placed below the T-tube can be torn out when the tube is removed. The integrity of the closure is tested by flushing saline through the T-tube. The long stem of the T-tube is brought out through a separate stab incision (shortest distance from the CBD to the exit site) and secured with 3-0 nonabsorbable monofilament sutures. A Jackson-Pratt drain is placed in Morison's pouch and is secured with 3-0 nonabsorbable monofilament sutures. The abdominal incision is closed as described above.

CHAPTER 25

Laparoscopic Cholecystectomy

EMBRYOLOGY AND ANATOMY See Chapter 24.

Operative Procedure

The preoperative preparations for laparoscopic cholecystectomy are essentially similar to those for open cholecystectomy (see Chapter 24).

POSITION The patient is placed in the supine position, and general anesthesia with endotracheal intubation is administered. To avoid possible inadvertent injury to the stomach or bladder, it is important to place a nasogastric tube and a Foley catheter. The patient is prepped and draped in the usual sterile fashion. Insufflation tubing, camera cables, and the suction tubing are all secured safely to the drapes. The laparoscopic camera is white balanced.

INCISION AND ESTABLISHMENT OF PNEUMOPERITONEUM A transverse skin-crease incision is made above the umbilicus, and blunt dissection of the subcutaneous tissue is performed to identify the linea alba. Using two towel clips, the operator grasps the skin and abdominal wall and inserts a Veres needle through the fascia into the peritoneal cavity. The tip of the Veres needle should be directed toward the feet of the patient to avoid inadvertent injury to the abdominal aorta. To confirm presence of the needle within the abdominal cavity, a drop test is performed: while the abdominal wall is pulled up with the towel clamps, a drop of saline is placed in the hub of the needle. The drop of saline should fall rapidly if the tip of the Veres needle is within the peritoneal cavity. Intra-abdominal insufflation is initiated, and the initial pressure reading should remain relatively low. High pressures early during insufflation indicate that the needle probably is improperly placed and should be repositioned or reinserted. If there is still concern regarding the position of the Veres needle, the surgeon should resort to an open technique using a Hasson cannula. In the open technique, after two stay sutures are placed using 0-0 absorbable sutures, the linea alba is incised and the peritoneal cavity entered. Under direct vision, the Hasson cannula with the blunt-tipped trocar is placed. If, however, insufflation is progressing well, the abdominal cavity should rise and be uniformly tympanitic upon percussion. The intra-abdominal pressure should be observed to rise gradually. Once the intra-abdominal pressure has reached about 15 mm Hg and approximately 2.5 to 3 L of CO_2 has been insufflated, the Veres needle is removed.

PLACEMENT OF PORTS   A 10-mm port is placed through the same transverse incision. The video camera is passed through the cannula to perform a careful laparoscopic examination to confirm its presence within the intra-abdominal cavity, to exclude any inadvertent injury, and to view the gallbladder. Next, three more ports need to be placed along the midline, midclavicular line, and anterior axillary line along a straight imaginary line that is equivalent to the traditional Kocher incision. The exact location of these ports, however, can be determined by pushing on the abdominal wall externally and then confirming that this location would be appropriate by viewing it with the video camera.

EXPOSURE AND OPERATIVE TECHNIQUE   Under direct vision, first a 10-mm port is placed in the midline approximately 5 to 6 cm below the xiphoid process. Next, 5-mm ports are placed in the midclavicular line and in the anterior axillary line. One of the fundamentals of safety in laparoscopic surgery is that every time an instrument is passed through the port it should be under direct vision; instruments should not be blindly inserted, to avoid inadvertent intra-abdominal injury.

Before the dissection begins, the patient is placed in the reverse Trendelenburg position and a ratcheted grasper is passed through the most lateral port to grasp the fundus of the gallbladder and retract it cephalad toward the right shoulder. Another ratcheted grasper is passed through the midclavicular port to grasp the infundibulum and is retracted laterally to place the cystic duct on tension. The peritoneal lining over the triangle of Calot is carefully incised using scissors. Some of the overlying adipose tissue can be bluntly teased to identify the cystic duct. With a right-angle dissector, the cystic duct is further dissected and its junction with the common bile duct clearly viewed. It is important to ensure that the junction of the gallbladder with the cystic duct is also confirmed to avoid inadvertent injury to the right hepatic duct. If it is difficult to identify the cystic duct–gallbladder junction, the peritoneal covering on each side of the gallbladder bed should be carefully divided. If the cystic duct–gallbladder junction is still not confidently identified, the procedure should be converted to an open cholecystectomy. Conversion to an open procedure should be considered not a defeat but a prudent decision by the surgeon.

If there are no plans to perform an operative cholangiogram, two proximal and two distal clips are placed and the cystic duct is sharply divided (Fig. 25–1A). With further blunt and sharp dissection in Calot's triangle, the cystic artery is identified and should be traced to the wall of the gallbladder. If the vessel is confirmed to be the cystic artery, it is secured with hemoclips and divided (see Fig. 25–1A). Next, the gallbladder is dissected from its bed. To achieve this, the infundibulum of the gallbladder is grasped adjacent to the hemoclips. While the gallbladder is rotated from side to side, the peritoneal covering and the loose areolar tissue are divided with hook electrocautery. As the dissection approaches the fundus of the gallbladder, cephalad retraction is lessened. The infundibulum is retracted, the gallbladder bed is inspected, and hemostasis is achieved. If any open biliary radicals are seen, they are secured with surgical clips.

Once the gallbladder is completely free from its hepatic bed, the camera is transferred to the infraxiphoid port and a retrievable bag is passed through the umbilical port (Fig. 25–1B). The gallbladder is pulled out through the umbilical wound. The umbilical incision may need to be extended if there is difficulty in extracting the distended gallbladder or if large stones are present. The right upper quadrant is thoroughly irrigated and any spilled bile or blood aspirated. If a drain is to be placed, it can be passed through the most lateral port and directed toward the subhepatic pouch of Morison under direct vision.

If a cholangiogram is to be performed, a single hemoclip is placed at the cystic duct–gallbladder junction. The cystic duct is carefully incised and the cholangiocatheter carefully placed within it. The cholangiocatheter is temporarily secured in place with a hemoclip. The cholangiogram can then be performed in the usual fashion. If the study is normal, cholecystectomy is performed as described above. Conversely, if stones are identified within the common bile duct, the surgeon must consider several options, including retrieving the stones by laparoscopic common bile duct exploration, proceeding with open common bile duct exploration, or completing the cholecystectomy and retrieving the stones via a postoperative endoscopic retrograde cholangiopancreatography. Before the abdomen is decompressed, the ports are removed under direct vision and the port sites are observed for any evidence of bleeding.

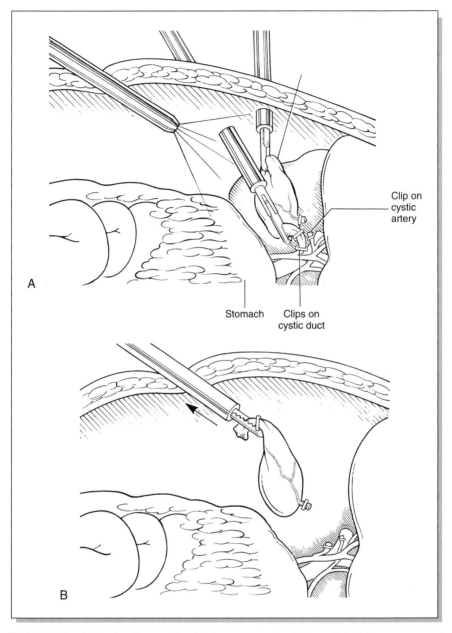

Clip on cystic artery

Stomach   Clips on cystic duct

A

B

FIGURE 25–1 *A,* The fundus and the Hartmann pouch of the gallbladder are grasped and retracted to visualize triangle of Calot. The cystic artery has been divided. Hemoclips have been placed across the cystic duct. *B,* The resected gallbladder is retrieved.

CLOSURE The fascial defects at the periumbilical and infraxiphoid locations are closed with figure-of-eight sutures using 0-0 absorbable sutures. The skin is approximated with subcuticular absorbable sutures and reinforced with Steri-Strips. Once the patient is awake in the recovery room, the nasogastric tube and the Foley catheter may be removed.

CHAPTER 26

Hepatic Resection

EMBRYOLOGY   The hepatic diverticulum arises from the caudal limit of the foregut from its ventral aspect and grows into the septum transversum. The hepatic diverticulum grows rapidly and starts to invade two sets of longitudinally placed vitelline and umbilical veins. The primary division of the liver into right and left sides is based on the invasion of hepatic tissue into right- and left-sided vitelline veins. The mesoderm of the septum, which extends from the liver to the ventral abdominal wall, becomes the falciform ligament with the umbilical vein present in its caudal margin. The mesoderm between the liver and the foregut forms the lesser omentum. The free edge of the lesser omentum contains the bile duct, which is the connection between the hepatic diverticulum and the foregut. The mesoderm on the surface of the liver differentiates into visceral peritoneum, except for the area in direct contact with the future diaphragm, which forms the bare area of the liver.

ANATOMY   The liver is the largest organ in the body, weighing approximately 1.5 kg. It is wedge shaped and lies predominantly in the right upper quadrant of the abdominal cavity. The liver is held in this position primarily by attachment of the hepatic veins to the inferior vena cava and by the peritoneal ligaments. The liver is attached to the anterior abdominal wall and the diaphragm by four distinctive ligaments: (1) the coronary ligament, which connects the posterior surface of the right hepatic lobe to the diaphragm with a superior and an inferior layer between that lies in the bare area of the liver; (2) the right triangular ligament, which is formed by fusion of the superior

153

and inferior layers of the coronary ligament; (3) the left triangular ligament, which connects the posterior surface of the left lobe of the liver to the
diaphragm; and (4) the sickle-shaped falciform ligament, which extends
from the diaphragm and anterior wall above the level of the umbilicus to
the surface of the liver, where it divides the left hepatic lobe into the left
lateral and left medial segments. The inferior free border of the falciform
ligament contains the ligamentum teres (obliterated umbilical vein).

A plane that extends from the gallbladder fossa to the inferior vena
cava, at approximately a 75-degree angle with the horizontal plane, is
called Cantlie's line. This line divides the liver into the right and left lobes
(Fig. 26–1). Further subdivisions of the liver are based on Couinaud
nomenclature. The two lobes are further subdivided into sectors on the
basis of the position of the major hepatic vein and their respective portal
pedicles. Each plane that divides the liver along the major hepatic vein is

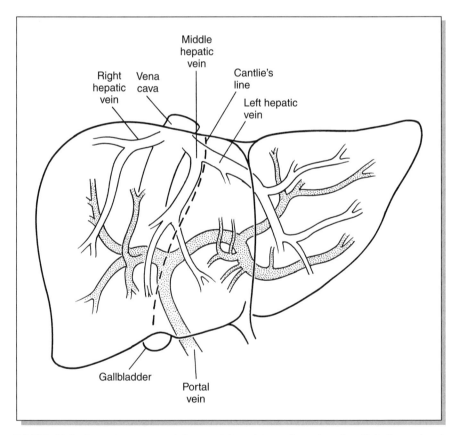

FIGURE 26–1 The distribution of the portal and hepatic veins. Cantlie's line extends
from the gallbladder to the inferior vena cava.

called a fissure. Though the term fissure is used, there is no groove to mark these planes in the intact liver, and thus Couinaud nomenclature refers to fissure as scissura.

The three major hepatic veins divide the liver into four sectors, namely, the left lateral, left medial, right anterior, and right posterior. The middle hepatic vein lies along the principal plane (the main fissure [scissura]), which extends from the gallbladder to the inferior vena cava. The left hepatic vein lies in the plane (left fissure [scissura]) formed by the falciform ligament. The plane that divides the right lobe into the posterior and anterior sectors contains the right hepatic vein (the right fissure [scissura]). These sectors are further subdivided into segments by a transverse plane along which lie the transversely placed right and left portal veins. This forms the basis for the Couinaud classification of liver anatomy, which divides the liver into eight independent segments, each with its own vascular inflow, outflow, and biliary drainage (Fig. 26–2). These segments are labeled numerically in a clockwise fashion, from 1 through 8, as shown in Figure 26–2. Segment 1 is also known as the caudate lobe, which lies adjacent to the inferior vena cava, and its venous drainage is directly into the vena cava.

The porta hepatis or the hilus of the liver is surrounded by a fibrous sheath, which invests the components of the pedicle. The hilum contains the main right and left hepatic ducts, the right and left branches of the hepatic artery, and the portal vein. The upper part of the free edge of the gastrohepatic ligament is attached to the margin of the porta hepatis. Also present in this region are hepatic lymph nodes.

In humans, the liver receives approximately 25% of the cardiac output. Approximately 75% is provided by portal venous blood flow and the remaining 25% by hepatic artery flow. The portal vein is formed by the union of the superior mesenteric vein and the splenic vein at the level of the second lumbar vertebra behind the head of pancreas. The portal vein enters the hilum of the liver and immediately divides into transversely placed right and left portal branches. The short right portal vein divides into posterior and inferior branches, each further dividing into superior and inferior branches that correspond to the segments described by Couinaud (see Fig. 26–1). The longer left portal vein divides into medial and lateral branches that further split into superior and inferior vessels, again corresponding with the hepatic segments. The left portal vein receives an attachment from the ligamentum venosum, which is a fibrous remnant of the embryonic ductus venosus.

The common hepatic artery arises from the celiac trunk, and after giving off the gastroduodenal and right gastric arteries, the proper hepatic artery courses toward the liver. This vessel subdivides into the right and left hepatic arteries that follow the portal vein branches. This is the standard hepatic arterial anatomy, although anatomic variations are common, with

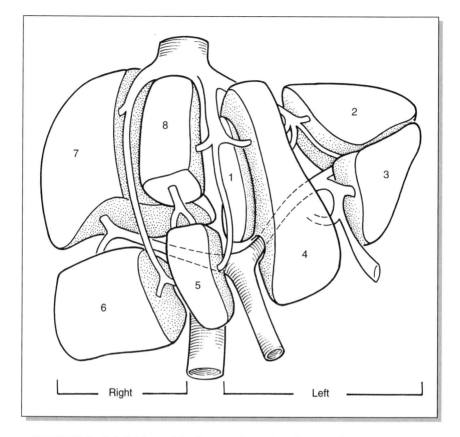

FIGURE 26–2 Subdivisions of the liver are based on Couinaud's nomenclature.

accessory or replaced hepatic arteries providing the sole source of arterial blood for a particular region within the liver. An aberrant artery is called an accessory hepatic artery if it supplies an area of the liver that also receives blood from a normal hepatic artery. Alternatively, it is known as a replaced hepatic artery if it is the only blood supply to such an area of the liver. An aberrant hepatic artery can arise from the aorta, the superior mesenteric artery, or the left gastric artery. Several authors have published the incidence of the anatomic variations based on radiologic or laparotomy findings (standard hepatic arterial anatomy, 58%–73%; replaced right hepatic artery from superior mesenteric artery, 12%–15%; replaced left hepatic artery from left gastric artery, 7%–10%; accessory right hepatic artery from superior mesenteric artery, 7%; accessory left hepatic artery from left gastric artery, 8%; common hepatic artery from superior mesenteric artery, 0–3%).

The venous drainage of the liver is through the three main hepatic veins and numerous very small veins that drain directly into the inferior vena cava (see Fig. 26–1). Of note, the middle hepatic vein can enter the inferior vena cava separately but more commonly joins the left hepatic vein to form a common trunk before joining the inferior vena cava. Because of this common anatomic variation, the operator should not ligate the middle or left hepatic vein before undertaking hepatic transection, which commonly can be performed safely with the right hepatic vein.

SPECIAL PREOPERATIVE PREPARATION   For any patient being considered for hepatic resection, it is imperative to assess hepatic function as well as the anatomic nature of the lesions, which would affect resectability. Hepatic function is assessed by liver function tests that include serum bilirubin, alkaline phosphatase, aspartate aminotransferase, alanine aminotransferase, and coagulation profile. Abnormalities of coagulation may require correction by transfusion of blood products along with administration of vitamin K. A review of hepatic imaging is crucial in determining the anatomic location of the hepatic space-occupying lesion and its relationship to the hepatic vein and portal vein. This assessment is best performed using computed tomography arterial portography. If the hepatic resection is being contemplated for malignant hepatic tumors, the patient should be assessed for extrahepatic metastasis by chest radiography or computed tomography of the chest, as necessary. Baseline carcinoembryonic antigen level and colonoscopy should be obtained if hepatectomy is being considered for colorectal metastases. Appropriate antibiotic prophylaxis is provided. Arrangements should also be made with the radiologist to perform intraoperative hepatic ultrasonography.

Operative Procedure

POSITION   The patient is placed in the supine position, and if necessary a log roll can be placed in the right flank. The patient undergoes general anesthesia with endotracheal intubation. A Swan-Ganz or a central venous catheter should be placed. To minimize blood loss during liver transection, the anesthesiologists should be requested to keep the central venous pressure at less than 5 cm H_2O. A nasogastric tube and Foley catheter are inserted, and sequential pneumatic compression devices are placed on the lower extremities. The patient's abdomen is prepped with an antiseptic solution and draped in the usual fashion.

INCISION   A chevron incision (bilateral subcostal incisions) is made approximately 3 to 4 cm below the costal margin. To maximize exposure, a vertical midline extension that extends to the xiphoid process is added to the chevron incision, thus converting it into the so-called Mercedes incision. A midline incision may be used particularly for limited resection or if the costal margin is narrow. The muscles of the anterior abdominal wall (as described for Kocher incision in Chapter 24) and linea alba are incised, and the abdominal cavity is entered.

EXPOSURE AND OPERATIVE TECHNIQUE A thorough exploration is performed to assess for the presence of peritoneal implants and suspicious regional adenopathy. If the procedure has been performed for colorectal metastases, lymph nodes in the porta hepatis should be biopsied, because the presence of metastatic disease would contraindicate hepatectomy.

In the absence of extrahepatic or disseminated disease, the procedure is begun by mobilizing the liver. First, division of the falciform ligament is extended to the hepatic veins posteriorly. The left triangular ligament is divided, with particular care taken not to injure the phrenic vessels. The phrenic vessels are carefully dissected, ligated in continuity with 2-0 silk sutures, and divided. Next, the right triangular ligament is divided to free the right lobe of the liver. After mobilization of the liver, intraoperative ultrasonography is performed to evaluate the relationship of the hepatic lesion to the hepatic vein and portal venous branches. In addition, it allows for a careful search to determine the presence of other intrahepatic tumor deposits that may need to be addressed.

If the hepatic mass is considered resectable, the next step involves encircling the contents of hepatoduodenal ligament with umbilical tape to allow inflow occlusion (Pringle maneuver). Controlling the major vascular structures aids in minimizing intraoperative blood loss. Intermittent vascular inflow occlusion is achieved using the Rummel tourniquet for 10 minutes with 5-minute intervals of reperfusion during parenchymal transection. For complex hepatic resections, some surgeons prefer to use total vascular exclusion. For this maneuver, the hepatoduodenal ligament and the suprahepatic and infrahepatic inferior venae cavae are isolated and Rummel-type tourniquets are placed. An initial trial exclusion must be undertaken for up to 5 minutes after adequately expanding intravascular volume to ensure that the procedure will be well tolerated. Clamps are applied in the following order: hepatoduodenal ligament, infrahepatic inferior vena cava, and suprahepatic inferior vena cava. The clamps are removed in the reverse order in which they were placed.

Right Hepatic Lobectomy

During right hepatic lobectomy, mobilization continues by division of the fine areolar tissue between the inferior vena cava and the liver. The liver is retracted anteriorly and to the left, thus allowing exposure to the multiple small, short hepatic veins between the inferior vena cava and segments 6 and 7, which are carefully ligated with 3-0 silk sutures.

Bleeding from very small veins can be controlled with hemoclips. As dissection proceeds more superiorly, the right hepatic vein will be encountered and should be carefully dissected and a vessel loop placed around it. Attempting to isolate the right hepatic vein without first freeing the liver from the inferior vena cava should be avoided. If feasible, the right hepatic vein can be divided between straight vascular clamps and oversewn with 3-0 polypropylene monofilament sutures; alternatively, transection can be performed with an endovascular stapling device (Fig. 26–3). This part of the dissection is crucial to avoid incurring hemorrhage by inadvertently tearing these small veins.

The exposure to the portal triad is improved by first performing a standard cholecystectomy. The peritoneal covering overlying the hepatic ligament is incised and dissected proximally toward the hilum of the liver. With the use of a Kittner dissector, the right hepatic artery and the right hepatic duct are dissected from the hilar plate. Vessel loops are placed

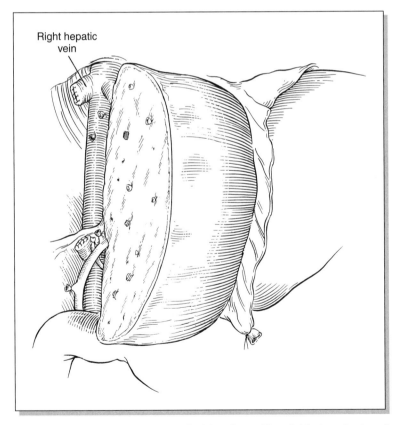

Right hepatic vein

FIGURE 26–3 Completion of right hepatic lobectomy. The divided and suture ligated right hepatic vein is seen.

around these structures. Careful medial retraction of these structures allows exposure of the portal vein. The right branch of the portal vein is carefully dissected and a vessel loop placed around it. The right hepatic bile duct is divided and also ligated with 2-0 silk suture ligatures. This is followed with division of the right hepatic artery, which is ligated with 2-0 silk suture ligatures. Proximally it is further secured with a 3-0 silk suture ligature. Next, the right portal vein is ligated in continuity and a 3-0 silk transfixion ligature is also applied. At this point a clear line of vascular demarcation along Cantlie's line will become evident, extending from the gallbladder back to the suprahepatic vena cava. Next, the liver is again retracted anteriorly and to the left, and the right hepatic vein is divided and suture ligated.

Hepatic parenchymal transection is commenced by first incising Glisson's capsule using electrocautery, just adjacent to the line of vascular demarcation. Intraoperative ultrasonography can again be used to delineate the location of the middle hepatic vein in relation to the plane of hepatic transection. The hepatic parenchyma can be transected in a variety of methods, including finger fracture, cautery, Kelly clamp dissection, an ultrasound aspirator, or sharply with a knife (guillotine technique). To reduce blood loss during hepatic transection, a Cooley vascular clamp is placed across the portal triad (Pringle maneuver). The anesthesiologist is informed once the clamp is placed and is asked to record the time. The surgeon and the assistant grasp the hepatic parenchyma with moist laparotomy pads adjacent to the line of transection. The liver is transected with a Kelly clamp. Intrahepatic venous, portal, and biliary radicals will be encountered and are secured with hemoclips. The hepatic parenchymal dissection is continued. Larger vascular and biliary radicals are suture ligated with 3-0 polypropylene monofilament sutures. The right branch of the portal vein is secured with continuous 3-0 polypropylene monofilament suture. Because the right hepatic vein and the short hepatic veins draining directly into the vena cava have already been secured, the resected lobe is simply removed. Hemostasis over the surface of the hepatic parenchyma is obtained with an argon beam laser coagulator (see Fig. 26–3). A moist laparotomy pad is placed over the surface. Any region staining yellow, indicating leaking biliary radicals, needs to be secured with either hemoclips or suture ligatures. The portal triad clamp is removed, and any further hemostasis is achieved.

Left Lateral Segmentectomy (Removal of Segments 2 and 3)

This procedure can be performed through the same incisions described in the previous section. The falciform ligament is divided between clamps and ligated with 2-0 silk sutures. The liver is mobilized in the standard fashion by incising the left triangular ligament, falciform ligament, and right triangular ligament. Intraoperative ultrasonography is performed, as described earlier. The peritoneal reflection overlying these structures within the hepatoduodenal ligament is incised and the left main hepatic artery identified. A vessel loop is placed around this vessel, making sure not to injure the right main hepatic artery. Next, the left branch of the portal vein and the left hepatic duct are dissected and a vessel loop placed around them. The left portal vein and the left hepatic artery are temporarily occluded with a soft Bulldog vascular clamp. The plane for resection of the lateral section of the left lobe is marked with electrocautery approximately 1 cm to the left of the falciform ligament. In this plane, only the terminal branches supplying the lateral segment of the left lobe are encountered. This avoids the danger of injuring the paraumbilicalis segment of the left portal vein and the paired portal venous branches (two superiorly and two inferiorly) to the medial segment of the left lobe (segment 4).

After incising Glisson's capsule, the surgeon and the assistant apply pressure on each side of the hepatic transection plane. The hepatic parenchyma can be divided in a variety of methods, as described in the previous section. The large ducts and vessels are individually ligated with 3-0 polypropylene monofilament sutures as they are encountered. Hepatic transection is continued posteriorly until the hepatic vein is visualized; it is divided and suture ligated with 3-0 polypropylene monofilament sutures. Vascular clamps are released, and the viability of the medial segment of the left lobe is assessed. The surface of the transected liver is electrocoagulated with an argon beam coagulator.

Left Hepatectomy

The incision, hepatic mobilization, and intraoperative ultrasound evaluation are as described in the previous sections. Next, the dissection proceeds at the hilum of the liver with identification of the left branch of the hepatic artery and portal vein, which are controlled with vessel loops. In a similar fashion the left hepatic vein is carefully dissected and controlled with a vessel loop. It is important to be aware that the middle hepatic vein unites with the left hepatic vein in 60% of the cases to form a common trunk before entering into the retrohepatic vena cava. The left branch of the portal vein and the hepatic artery are clamped, producing a line of demarcation along the main fissure (scissura). The position of the middle hepatic vein in relation to the line of demarcation can be confirmed intraoperatively with ultrasonography.

Dissection begins by incision of the Glisson capsule just to the left of Cantlie's line. The gallbladder may need to be removed if the dissection is very close to its surface. The left branch of the hepatic artery and the left hepatic duct are ligated with 2-0 silk sutures and divided. This exposes the left branch of the portal vein, which is next divided between clamps and suture ligated with continuous 3-0 polypropylene monofilament sutures. The hepatic parenchyma is transected in the manner described earlier, and the plane of dissection can be confirmed with intraoperative ultrasonography. Surgeons should be careful in keeping to the left of the middle hepatic vein to avoid inadvertent injury. Once the vena cava is reached, the left hepatic vein is identified, clamped, divided, and suture ligated with 3-0 polypropylene monofilament sutures (Fig. 26–4). Hemostasis is secured as described earlier. Biliary radical leaks should be controlled with suture ligation using 3-0 polypropylene monofilament sutures or hemoclips. Hemostasis is secured with an argon beam laser coagulator.

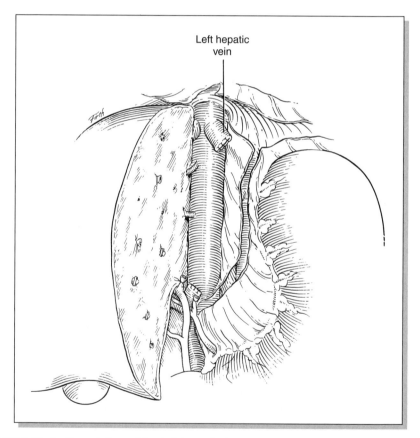

FIGURE 26–4 Completion of the left hepatic lobectomy. The divided and ligated left hepatic vein is shown.

Nonanatomic Liver Resection (Wedge Resection, Limited Resection)

Wedge resections involve removal of liver tissue without reference to segmental anatomy (i.e., nonanatomic resections). Even though a wedge resection of the liver is contemplated, it is imperative to mobilize the liver and perform intraoperative ultrasonography to exclude the presence of other hepatic space-occupying lesions. The lesser omentum is opened, which will allow placement of a vascular clamp to perform the Pringle maneuver. The proposed site of hepatic resection around the lesion is marked with electrocautery, keeping at least 1 cm of margin. The Glisson capsule is incised, and hepatic parenchyma is easily dissected with any of the previously described methods. Biliary radicals and hepatic vasculature are identified, secured with hemoclips, and divided. Vessels and bile ducts larger than 2 mm are ligated in continuity with 3-0 silk sutures and divided. Hemostasis is secured at the raw surface of the liver with an argon beam laser coagulator.

CLOSURE The peritoneum and posterior rectus sheath are approximated with 1-0 polypropylene monofilament sutures. The external oblique fascia and the linea alba (at the midline extension) are closed with 1-0 polypropylene monofilament sutures.

CHAPTER 27

Biliary Drainage Procedures

PREOPERATIVE PREPARATION Preoperative preparation is essentially similar to that described for a cholecystectomy (see Chapter 24). Surgical biliary procedures are primarily performed for decompression in the presence of obstruction within the extrahepatic biliary system. A variety of methods are described, and their use will depend on the site of obstruction; the mode of presentation, namely whether it is chronic or acute; and the suspected underlying pathology.

Operative Procedure

POSITION The patient is placed in the supine position on an operating table that allows the surgeon to perform operative cholangiography.

INCISION The incisions most commonly used for exploration of the bile ducts are the subcostal (Kocher) incision and the upper midline incision. The choice between these two incisions depends on surgeon preference and other structures that may need to be exposed.

Cholecystostomy

In high-risk patients cholecystotomy may be performed percutaneously by an interventional radiologist. This procedure, however, is performed very rarely and only under special circumstances, either because of the poor general condition of the patient or as a result of associated severe cirrhosis that may make cholecystectomy hazardous. However, if there is evidence of either perforation or gangrenous cholecystitis, cholecystectomy is preferable.

Once the peritoneal cavity is entered, a careful exploration is performed. Moist laparotomy pads are placed in Morison's pouch to avoid any spillage of bile. A purse-string suture using 2-0 silk is placed at the fundus of the gallbladder. A second purse-string suture using 2-0 silk is placed 1 cm away. A trocar is placed through the fundus of the gallbladder to empty its contents. Once the gallbladder is decompressed, often gallstones can be palpated at the neck; these can easily be milked out or removed using Desjardins forceps. The trocar is removed, and through the same stab incision a 20 Fr Foley or a Malecot catheter is placed into the gallbladder. If a Foley catheter is used, the balloon is inflated with 5 to 10 mL of distilled water. The purse-string suture is tied down securely. To seal the fundus of the gallbladder and to prevent bile leak, the second purse-string suture is snugly tied down. The long end of the Foley is brought out through a separate stab incision in the anterior abdominal wall and secured with 3-0 nonabsorbable monofilament sutures. A 10-mm Jackson-Pratt drain is left in the hepatorenal fossa to drain potential bile leaks.

Transduodenal Sphincteroplasty

Sphincteroplasty is a useful procedure where there is impaction of a gallstone in the ampulla of Vater or fibrous stricture of the sphincter of Oddi. Initially, the common bile duct is exposed just proximal to the first part of the duodenum. Next, a Kocher maneuver is performed. Two 4-0 silk stay sutures are placed on the anterior wall of the common bile duct, and a longitudinal incision is made as close to the duodenum as possible, in case a choledochoduodenostomy becomes necessary. Through the choledochotomy, a Bakes dilator is passed to the level of the ampulla. The site where the tip of the Bakes dilator is palpated can be used to center the longitudinal incision on the anterior duodenal wall. By placing stay sutures at the edges, the operator can retract the duodenal wall outward to improve exposure. The direction in which the Bakes dilator lies provides a clue to the course of the distal common bile duct. Keeping this in mind, two stay sutures using 4-0 silk are placed at the level of the ampulla, and an oblique incision at approximately the 11 o'clock position is made. If there is an impacted stone, this should be removed from below. A rush of bile may be seen emerging through the sphincterotomy. After this initial incision of the ampulla, graduated Bakes dilators can be readily passed from above through the sphincter and into the duodenum. Any fine biliary stones or debris can be flushed from above using saline irrigations through a red Robinson catheter. The sphincterotomy should be approximately 1.5 cm and can be extended with Pott scissors. Once the operator is satisfied with the length of the sphincterotomy, interrupted simple sutures using 4-0 absorbable sutures are placed at the two edges of the sphincterotomy. To avoid the possibility of bile leak, a figure-of-eight suture is placed at the apex of the sphincterotomy. The duodenotomy is closed in the usual fashion in two layers with an inner continuous Connell suture using 3-0 absorbable sutures and an outer seromuscular layer of interrupted 3-0 silk Lembert sutures. Finally, a 10-mm Jackson-Pratt drain is placed in the hepatorenal fossa.

Choledochoduodenostomy

For this procedure to be performed, the diameter of the common bile duct must be greater than 1.5 cm because the anastomosis between the common bile duct and the duodenum should be at least 2.5 cm in diameter to allow free drainage of bile. The peritoneal covering over the common bile duct is carefully cleared, using blunt dissection with a Kittner, avoiding any dissection on the lateral aspect because this can injure the delicate blood supply. A Kocher maneuver is required before performing a tension-free anastomosis. Two stay sutures using 4-0 silk are placed on the anterior surface of the common bile duct. A longitudinal incision, measuring approximately 1.5 to 2.0 cm, is made in the common bile duct as close to the duodenum as possible. Next, after placement of two stay sutures, a transverse incision is made in the first part of the duodenum adjacent to the common bowel duct. A one-layer anastomosis is sufficient and can be constructed with a single layer of interrupted 3-0 absorbable sutures. A 10-mm Jackson-Pratt drain is placed in the hepatorenal (Morison's pouch) fossa.

Choledochojejunostomy/Hepaticojejunostomy

When an anastomosis between the bowel and the common hepatic or common bile duct is needed, the jejunum becomes the preferable conduit. The common bile duct is identified and its anterior surface dissected in preparation for the anastomosis. The ligament of Treitz is identified, and 15 cm distal to this point, the jejunum is transected using a GIA linear stapler. The peritoneum lining over the mesentery is incised with electrocautery, and at least two or three of the vascular arcades are divided and ligated to allow the distal segment of the jejunum to reach the bile duct. An opening is made in the nonvascular portion of the transverse mesocolon, and the distal jejunal limb is passed through this defect toward the common bile duct. The anastomosis can be side to end, end to side, or end to end. However, an end (common bile duct)-to-side (jejunum) anastomosis is preferred, and it requires transection of the common bile or common hepatic duct. A one-layer anastomosis is constructed by approximating mucosa to mucosa with simple interrupted 4-0 absorbable sutures (Fig. 27–1). Just before the anterior layer of the anastomosis is completed (Fig. 27–2A), a T-tube is placed as a stent and the longer limb is brought out through the bile duct. If the anastomosis is constructed for a bile duct injury in the acute setting, the common bile duct is generally of normal caliber, and therefore the anastomosis needs to be protected with a T-tube (Fig. 27–2B). To avoid any tension on the anastomosis, the jejunum is secured to the adjacent liver capsule or the adjacent peritoneal lining of the lesser omentum. Finally, a hand-sewn end-to-side jejunojejunostomy is performed about 60 cm from the choledochojejunostomy with an inner

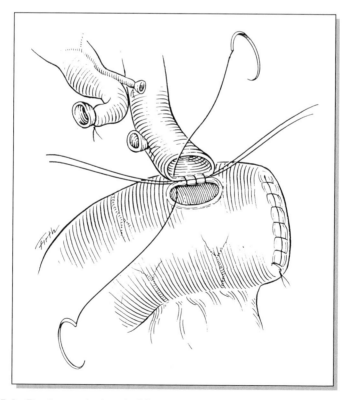

FIGURE 27–1 The transected end of the common bile duct is sutured to the side of a jejunal limb.

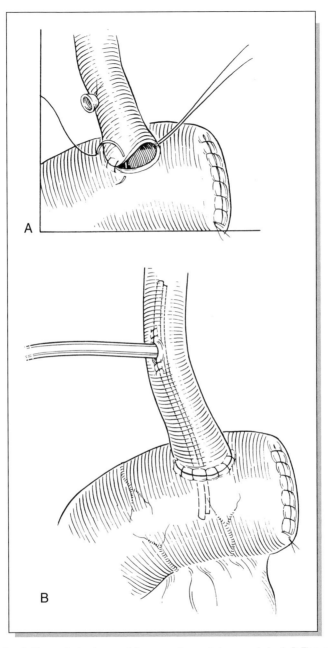

FIGURE 27–2 *A,* The anterior layer of the anastomosis is completed. *B,* The anastomosis is protected with a T-tube as a stent.

continuous layer of 3-0 absorbable sutures and an outer layer of 3-0 silk Lembert sutures. A few interrupted sutures between the mesocolon and the jejunal limb are placed to close the defect in the mesocolon. A 10-mm Jackson-Pratt drain is placed in the right upper quadrant.

CLOSURE   The abdominal incision is closed in the usual fashion.

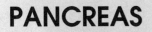

PANCREAS

CHAPTER 28

Pancreatico-duodenectomy (Whipple Procedure)

EMBRYOLOGY The ectodermal epithelium of the duodenum gives rise to two pancreatic buds. In the ventral mesentery is the ventral pancreatic bud, and opposite it is the larger dorsal pancreatic bud lying within the dorsal mesoderm. Because of the retroperitoneal location of the duodenum, the dorsal pancreas comes to lie on the posterior body wall in the retroperitoneal position and within the concavity of the duodenum. The ventral pancreas comes to lie adjacent to the larger dorsal bud due to the rotation of the stomach and the migration of the liver toward the dorsal body wall.

Once both the ventral and dorsal pancreas lie in the C-shaped concavity of the duodenum, they fuse. The ventral bud forms the uncinate process, whereas the bulk of the pancreas is derived from the dorsal bud. The main pancreatic duct (duct of Wirsung) is formed by the distal part of the dorsal duct and the entire ventral pancreatic duct. The proximal part of the dorsal pancreatic duct either obliterates or persists as the accessory pancreatic duct (duct of Santorini).

ANATOMY The pancreas is a retroperitoneal organ that measures approximately 15 cm in length and weighs approximately 80 g. It is a soft and lobulated organ that extends from the C-loop of the duodenum to the hilum of the spleen. For descriptive purposes, the pancreas is divided into a head, neck, body, and tail.

The head of the pancreas lies within the C-loop of the duodenum and inferiorly bears an uncinate process that passes to the left behind the superior mesenteric vessels. This relationship is important when encountering tumors in this region and during their resection while performing a pancreaticoduodenectomy. The neck of the pancreas lies at the level of the portal vein and origin of the superior mesenteric artery. The body is a triangular segment of pancreas that travels upward and to the left. Finally, the tail of the pancreas travels upward within the splenorenal ligament to reach the splenic hilum.

There are important anatomic relationships to the pancreas that have surgical relevance. These are described according to the different segments of the pancreas. The superior, lateral, and inferior borders of the head of the pancreas are embraced by the C-loop of the duodenum. Structures that lie anterior to the pancreatic head include the pylorus and the transverse colon. Posteriorly, the head is near the inferior vena cava and the common bile duct. The uncinate process of the head of the pancreas is crossed anteriorly by the superior mesenteric vessels. The neck lies in front of the origin of the portal vein; lying anterior to this are the pylorus and the gastroduodenal artery. Immediately above the body of the pancreas is the celiac axis; the tortuous splenic artery runs along its upper border. The splenic vein lies along the posterior surface of the body of the pancreas. At the inferior border the two leaves of the transverse mesocolon are attached. The anterior surface of the body of the pancreas is covered by the peritoneum of the lesser sac.

The main pancreatic duct (the duct of Wirsung) traverses the main body of the pancreas and joins the common bile duct, entering the posteromedial aspect of the second part of the duodenum at the ampulla of Vater, which is surrounded by the sphincter of Oddi. The accessory pancreatic duct (the duct of Santorini) drains the upper part of the head of the pancreas and opens approximately 2 cm proximal to the main duct.

The arterial supply of the pancreas is derived from the branches of the celiac axis and the superior mesenteric artery. The head of the pancreas and the C-loop of the duodenum are intimately supplied by the pancreaticoduodenal arcades. The superior and inferior pancreaticoduodenal arteries are derived from the gastroduodenal artery and the middle colic arteries, respectively. Both the superior and inferior pancreaticoduodenal arteries branch into anterior and posterior branches, which create an arterial arcade around the head of the pancreas. Ligation of these vessels during resection of the head of the pancreas would lead to duodenal necrosis because the head of the pancreas and the C-loop of the duodenum share this blood supply. Consequently, during the Whipple procedure both the head of the pancreas and the C-loop of the duodenum must be resected.

The splenic artery provides numerous branches to the pancreas, including the dorsal pancreatic artery. There are numerous collaterals between the small branches derived from the splenic artery and the dorsal and transverse pancreatic arteries. Therefore, ligation of the splenic artery does not require splenectomy, but ligation of the splenic vein does.

The venous drainage of the pancreas parallels the arterial supply and includes the portal, the splenic, and both the superior and inferior mesenteric veins. As indicated earlier, the superior mesenteric vein and the splenic vein join behind the neck of the pancreas to form the portal vein. The lymphatic drainage is along the lymph nodes situated adjacent to the arteries that supply the pancreas. These lymph nodes eventually drain into the celiac and superior mesenteric lymph nodes.

PREOPERATIVE PREPARATION In addition to the routine assessment of the cardiac, respiratory, and renal function of the patient, it is vital to review the high-resolution spiral computed tomography scan of the abdomen and pelvis with 3-mm cuts through the pancreas. Attention is paid to the presence of local invasion of adjacent vessels, particularly the superior mesenteric vessels and the portal vein. Major vessel occlusion and/or encasement, liver metastases, or enlarged celiac axis lymph nodes are ominous signs of incurable disease. Chest x-ray is also reviewed. If the patient is noted to have sepsis related to jaundice, preoperative biliary drainage may be advisable. Preoperative tissue diagnosis of a pancreatic mass is unnecessary if it is considered resectable by computed tomographic findings.

Operative Procedure

POSITION The patient is placed in the supine position. General anesthesia is achieved with endotracheal intubation. A nasogastric tube and a Foley catheter and sequential pneumatic compression devices are placed. Perioperative antibiotics are administered. The abdomen is shaved, prepped, and draped in the usual manner. The procedure begins initially with a diagnostic laparoscopy. If there is no overt evidence of peritoneal, omental, or liver metastasis, the surgeon can proceed with exploratory laparotomy.

INCISION A right subcostal incision extending toward the left side is made and carried down through the subcutaneous tissue and anterior rectus sheath. The rectus muscle and the posterior rectus sheath are divided with electrocautery.

EXPOSURE AND OPERATIVE TECHNIQUE The ligamentum teres is divided between clamps and ligated with 2-0 silk. The falciform ligament is divided to the level of the inferior vena cava, thus allowing bimanual palpation of the liver. A thorough exploration is again undertaken, with particular attention to the presence of any peritoneal implants or periaortic or celiac axis lymphadenopathy. Liberal biopsies of suspicious peritoneal implants and enlarged lymph nodes that are beyond the limits of normal resection should be performed, because these contraindicate resection. The transverse colon is lifted, and the mesocolon is palpated just medial to the ligament of Treitz, because invasion in this region would involve the middle colic vessels, thus necessitating segmental colon resection.

Once evidence of distant metastasis has been excluded, the next step is to determine whether the primary tumor is resectable; this is done by excluding invasion of the adjacent vascular structures (inferior vena cava, superior mesenteric vessels, portal vein, and aorta) by the tumor. Adequate exposure is essential, and the use of a self-retaining abdominal retractor facilitates the procedure. Mobilization of the right colon and the hepatic flexure is begun to provide access to the second part of the duodenum. A wide Kocher maneuver is performed, and the duodenum and pancreas are elevated off the inferior vena cava until the left border of the abdominal aorta can be palpated. The Kocher maneuver is extended by continuing mobilization of the third portion of the duodenum until the superior mesenteric vein is encountered. The gastrocolic ligament is divided just inferior to the gastroepiploic arcade to gain access to the lesser sac. To improve access to the anterior surface of the pancreatic head, the right gastroepiploic vein is divided as it crosses the neck of the pancreas to enter the superior mesenteric vein. The middle colic vein is identified and followed down to its confluence with the superior mesenteric vein, which was previously identified during the extensive Kocher maneuver. The anterior surface of the superior mesenteric vein is dissected under direct vision. Using a Cushing vein retractor, the neck of the pancreas is lifted, and entering this avascular plane, the superior mesenteric vein is traced proximally to its confluence with the portal vein.

Once sufficient inferior dissection has been performed, the superior aspect of the dissection is commenced. This portion of the procedure is greatly facilitated by first performing a cholecystectomy. The peritoneal reflection over the hepatoduodenal ligament is carefully opened, and the common bile duct and common hepatic artery are carefully dissected and vessel loops are placed around them. The adipose and nodal tissues in this region are dissected toward the specimen. The gastroduodenal artery is identified and ligated in continuity to facilitate access to the portal vein at the superior aspect of the pancreas. Exposing the interface between the bile duct and the portal vein facilitates the process of adequately assessing resectability, and this can be achieved by dividing the common hepatic duct.

Even if the tumor is unresectable, the divided common hepatic duct can be used to construct the choledochojejunostomy. Thus, division of both the gastroduodenal artery and the common hepatic duct untethers the first portion of the duodenum, which can now be retracted, thus allowing further dissection, under direct vision, of the anterior surface of the portal vein from the superior aspect. Such exposure will eliminate the need for blind finger dissection to assess the plane between the neck of the pancreas and the portal vein. Palpation behind the head of the pancreas is necessary to determine if the tumor has invaded the uncinate process, the posterior aspect of the portal vein, or the superior mesenteric artery (Fig. 28–1).

At this point if there is no evidence of encroachment of the tumor to the major regional vessels, a decision to proceed with formal resection is made. To ensure adequate regional lymphadenectomy, tissues over the

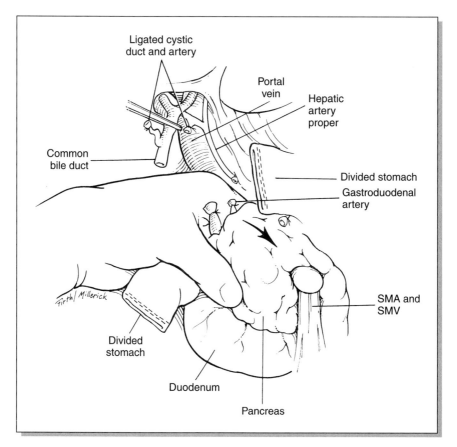

FIGURE 28–1 The gastric antrum, common hepatic duct, and gastroduodenal artery have been divided. To assess resectability, the surgeon is performing careful digital exploration by placing the index finger between the pancreatic neck and the portal vein. SMA, superior mesenteric artery; SMV, superior mesenteric vein.

medial border of the kidney, the right renal vein, and the inferior vena cava must be included en bloc with the specimen. In a similar fashion, the lymphatic tissue overlying the hepatoduodenal ligament and adjacent to the superior mesenteric vein is swept toward the specimen. If the common hepatic duct has not been divided during the process of assessing resectability, it can be done at this stage. Two 5-0 Prolene stay sutures are placed on the anterolateral aspect of the bile duct before its division. The distal end can be occluded with a large hemoclip. Next, if a standard pancreaticoduodenectomy is to be performed, the distal part of the stomach is mobilized and transected with a GIA-90 linear stapler.

Next, the duodenojejunal flexure is located and dissected free from the retroperitoneum by dividing the ligament of Treitz (Fig. 28–2). Approximately 10 to 15 cm distal to the duodenojejunal flexure, the peritoneal lining is scored with electrocautery and the vessels within the mesentery are divided and ligated with 2-0 silk sutures. The small bowel

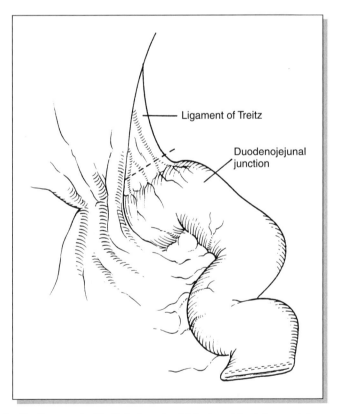

FIGURE 28–2 The ligament of Treitz is sharply divided and the jejunum is transected with a GIA-60 linear stapler.

is divided with a GIA-60 linear stapler (see Fig. 28–2). Mobilization of the small bowel is continued, and it is passed beneath the superior mesenteric vessels toward the patient's right side.

The next step is to transect the neck of the pancreas, which is begun by first placing figure-of-eight 2-0 silk sutures approximately 1 cm apart at the superior and inferior aspect of the pancreas to control bleeding from the pancreaticoduodenal arteries. To avoid injury to the underlying superior mesenteric vein and portal vein, a narrow malleable or a one-fourth–inch Penrose drain is placed and the pancreas is divided with a no. 15 scalpel between the previously placed hemostatic sutures. Bleeding from the specimen side of the pancreas can be controlled with hemoclips, whereas that from the body of the pancreas is achieved with suture ligatures using 3-0 silk.

The cut end of the head of the pancreas and the divided stomach is retracted toward the patient's right. This exposes the anterior surface of the superior mesenteric vein and portal vein. Several small vessels draining directly from the head of the pancreas into the superior mesenteric vein on the right side are encountered and are carefully isolated, ligated in continuity with 3-0 silk, and divided. The uncinate process is divided either with a TA-55 stapler or between clamps and then ligated carefully with 3-0 silk suture ligatures. Before dividing the uncinate process, it is wise to check that there is no major anomalous hepatic artery originating from the superior mesenteric artery. The specimen contains the gastric antrum, duodenum, head of the pancreas, distal common bile duct, and proximal jejunum and is sent to the pathology lab (Fig. 28–3). Frozen sections of the margins of the bile duct, pancreatic body, and uncinate process are obtained.

The pancreatic duct is identified using a lacrimal probe. In preparation for the anastomoses, the jejunal limb is passed through a defect in the transverse mesocolon. To restore gastrointestinal continuity, pancreaticojejunostomy is performed, followed by the choledochojejunostomy 10 cm distally. Approximately 15 cm distal to the choledochojejunostomy, the gastrojejunostomy is performed.

The pancreaticojejunal anastomosis can be created in a variety of ways depending on size of the pancreatic duct and the consistency of the pancreas. If the pancreatic duct is enlarged, usually a pancreaticojejunal duct–to–mucosa anastomosis is performed. First, a posterior layer of interrupted 3-0 silk is placed between the pancreatic capsule and the jejunum. Next, a small enterotomy is made in the adjacent jejunum. At least four interrupted duct-to-mucosal sutures are placed using 5-0 polypropylene and then tagged with fine Halsted mosquito clamps. A no. 5 Fr stent is passed into the pancreatic duct and then brought out through the jejunum, via a small incision, before these sutures are tied down. Finally, the anterior layer of sutures is placed between the jejunum and pancreatic

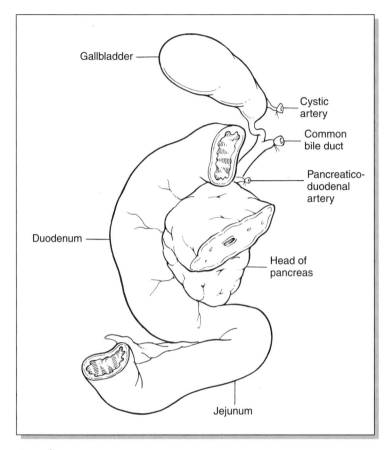

Gallbladder

Cystic artery

Common bile duct

Pancreatico-duodenal artery

Duodenum

Head of pancreas

Jejunum

FIGURE 28–3 The resected specimen contains the gastric antrum, duodenum, head of the pancreas, distal common bile duct, and proximal jejunum.

tissue using 3-0 silk. Approximately 10 cm distally, an enterotomy is made within the same jejunal loop, and an end-to-side choledochojejunal anastomosis is performed using interrupted 3-0 nonabsorbable monofilament sutures. An additional anterior layer of seromuscular sutures may be used.

If the common hepatic duct is of small caliber, it can be stented with a T-tube. The third anastomosis is then performed between the stomach and the jejunum in two layers with inner continuous 3-0 absorbable sutures and outer interrupted Lembert-type sutures using 3-0 silk. Approximately 15 to 20 cm distal to the gastrojejunostomy a standard feeding jejunostomy is placed. Using two separate stab incisions in the right upper quadrant, 10-mm Jackson-Pratt drains are placed adjacent to the pancreaticojejunostomy and choledochojejunostomy to drain potential anastomotic leaks. If a T-tube has been used to stent the choledochojejunostomy, this is brought out through a separate stab incision in the right upper quadrant. The defect in the mesocolon is closed by means of continuous or interrupted 3-0 absorbable sutures. The operative area is thoroughly irrigated with warm saline.

If a pylorus-preserving pancreaticoduodenectomy is to be performed, the first part of the duodenum is carefully mobilized from the head of the pancreas and divided approximately 2 cm distal to the pylorus using a GIA-55 stapling device. After the pancreatic tumor has been resected, the pancreaticojejunostomy and the choledochojejunostomy are performed as described earlier, followed by an end-to-side duodenojejunostomy.

CLOSURE   The abdominal wall is closed in layers using 1-0 monofilament absorbable sutures. The drains are secured to the skin with 3-0 nylon.

CHAPTER 29

Distal Pancreatectomy

EMBRYOLOGY AND ANATOMY   See Chapter 28.

PREOPERATIVE PREPARATION   Preoperative preparation should essentially be similar to that for pancreaticoduodenectomy. If the pancreatic resection is to be performed for a functioning neuroendocrine tumor, the clinical syndrome resulting from excess hormone production may need to be controlled before surgery. Administration of octreotide has been particularly useful in these situations. Alternatively, specific blocking agents such as omeprazole for gastrinoma and diazoxide for insulinoma can also be used. Because splenectomy is performed as part of distal pancreatectomy, the patient should receive prophylactic Pneumovax vaccination. Broad-spectrum antibiotics are administered perioperatively.

ANESTHESIA   General anesthesia with endotracheal intubation is instituted. A nasogastric tube, Foley catheter, and sequential pneumatic compression devices are placed over the lower extremities.

Operative Procedure

POSITION   The patient is placed in the supine position.

INCISION   A long upper midline incision or a bilateral subcostal incision can be made.

EXPOSURE AND OPERATIVE TECHNIQUE Upon entering the abdomen, a thorough exploration is performed to detect possible metastatic disease. To expose the anterior surface of the pancreas, the lesser sac is approached by serially dividing the gastrocolic and gastrosplenic ligaments and elevating the stomach cephalad. Within the gastrosplenic ligament, the short gastric vessels are divided and ligated. On the gastric side, the short gastric vessels are suture ligated with 3-0 silk. The transverse colon is displaced downward into the lower abdomen to improve exposure. With electrocautery, the peritoneal covering at the superior and inferior borders of the pancreas is divided. This is best performed by carefully opening planes with fine Schnidt clamps and dividing the tissue with electrocautery.

Mobilization of the pancreas is theoretically best performed from the left to the right side. The spleen is retracted medially, which places the splenorenal ligament under tension. This ligament is divided, and the spleen is drawn forward together with the tail of the pancreas, thus opening the retropancreatic plane. Having freed the superior and inferior borders of the pancreas earlier, the operator can mobilize the pancreas to a level proximal to the tumor (Fig. 29–1). Here the splenic vein and artery are carefully dissected with a right-angle Mixter clamp and ligated in continuity with 2-0 silk. The splenic vessels are ligated in continuity and divided. The vessels are further secured with 3-0 silk transfixion ligatures.

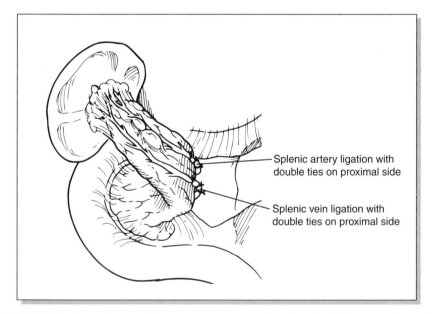

Splenic artery ligation with
double ties on proximal side

Splenic vein ligation with
double ties on proximal side

FIGURE 29–1 The spleen and the pancreas are mobilized medially. The splenic vessels are ligated in continuity and divided.

Before transecting the pancreas sutures, the operator ligates the superior and inferior pancreaticoduodenal vessels with 3-0 silk transfixion sutures. The pancreas is divided with electrocautery. Bleeding is controlled with figure-of-eight sutures using 3-0 silk in the pancreatic substance. The anterior and posterior borders of the pancreas are approximated with interrupted mattress sutures using 3-0 silk.

The abdomen is irrigated with warm saline. Through a separate stab incision, a 10-mm Jackson-Pratt drain is placed adjacent to the cut end of the body of the pancreas. The drain is secured with 3-0 nylon.

CLOSURE　The anterior abdominal wall is closed in layers using 1-0 absorbable polydioxanone. The skin is approximated with staples.

SPLEEN

CHAPTER 30

Splenectomy

EMBRYOLOGY   The spleen develops from a mass of mesenchymal cells located within the dorsal mesentery. As it enlarges it becomes lobulated and projects into the greater sac. The notch on the anterior border of the spleen is the remnant of this fetal lobulation. Embryologic development of the spleen assists in understanding of the ligament attachments present in the adult. As the stomach rotates, the left surface of the dorsal mesentery fuses with the posterior body wall over the left kidney; this explains the development of the splenorenal ligament. Dorsal mesentery between the spleen and the stomach represents the gastrosplenic ligament.

ANATOMY   The spleen is an ovoid lymphoid organ that resides in the left upper quadrant. It weighs approximately 200 g and measures approximately 12 cm long, 8 cm wide, and 4 cm thick. The long axis of the spleen lies along the tenth rib. The spleen has two surfaces: the outer diaphragmatic surface and the medial visceral surface that bears the hilum. The anterior border has a notch that can be palpable when the spleen is enlarged. The spleen has several ligaments, and their names indicate their connections. The splenorenal ligament contains the splenic vessels and the tail of the pancreas. The gastrosplenic ligament contains several short gastric vessels. Some of the other minor ligaments surrounding the spleen include the splenocolic ligament, the splenophrenic ligament, the pancreaticosplenic ligament, and the phrenosplenic fold, which lies anterior to the gastrosplenic ligament.

The blood supply of the spleen originates from the splenic artery, which is a branch of the celiac axis. The splenic artery is a very tortuous vessel that runs along the upper border of the pancreas to reach the splenic hilum, where it divides into several branches. The venous drainage of the spleen flows into the splenic vein. The splenic vein lies along the posterior surface of the pancreas and joins the superior mesenteric vein to form the portal vein. The lymphatic drainage of the spleen is along the splenic artery via the superior pancreatic nodes to the celiac group of para-aortic nodes.

The incidence of accessory spleens varies from 10% to 30%. Most of these are present at the splenic hilum or near the tail of the pancreas. However, accessory spleens can be found in other areas such as the omentum, the splenocolic ligament, and along the path of the splenic artery. In approximately two thirds of patients only one accessory spleen is present, and in another 15% to 20% two such accessory spleens are present.

Operative Procedure

POSITION The patient is placed in a supine position. After induction of anesthesia and endotracheal intubation, a nasogastric tube and Foley catheter are placed. A prophylactic dose of antibiotics is administered, and external pneumatic compression devices are placed on the lower extremities.

INCISION The incision used depends on the size of the spleen, whether emergency access to the abdomen is required, and whether there is an underlying coagulation disorder. In emergent cases and in patients with a large spleen, a midline incision is preferred. Small spleens can be accessed via a left subcostal incision.

EXPOSURE AND OPERATIVE TECHNIQUE A thorough exploration of the abdomen is performed, with particular attention directed to identifying accessory spleens and palpating the gallbladder for calculi. A self-retaining Balfour retractor is then placed, and the assistant lifts the left costal margin with a large Richardson retractor to expose the structures in the left upper quadrant.

The spleen is gently grasped with the palm of the hand and displaced medially toward the incision. This places the avascular lateral peritoneal attachments (splenorenal and splenophrenic ligaments) under tension, and they are incised with Metzenbaum scissors or electrocautery (Fig. 30–1). This dissection usually does not lead to significant bleeding unless collaterals from existing portal hypertension are present, in which case they must be ligated. Division of the lateral peritoneal ligaments allows the spleen to be drawn farther toward the surgeon. Dry laparotomy pads are placed in the splenic bed for hemostasis and to facilitate elevation

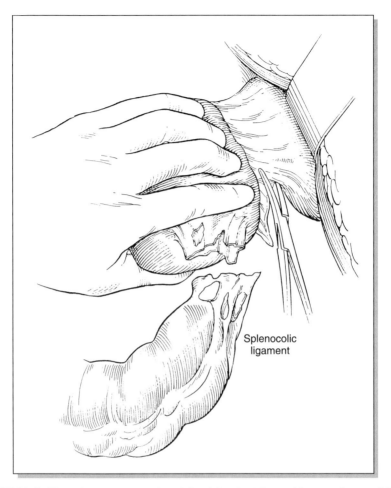

FIGURE 30–1 The spleen is grasped and the lateral peritoneal ligaments are divided. The splenocolic ligaments have been divided to release the splenic flexure.

and mobilization of the medially rotated spleen. At the lower portion the splenocolic ligament is divided, thus releasing the splenic flexure (see Fig. 30–1). The splenic artery is identified, carefully dissected, doubly ligated with 0 silk, and then divided. Proximally, it is also transfixed with 3-0 silk suture ligatures. If the patient requires platelet transfusions, they can be administered at this stage. The splenic vein is similarly isolated, doubly ligated, and divided, and the proximal end is transfixed with 3-0 silk suture ligatures. Both vessels should be ligated close to the hilum to avoid injury to the tail of the pancreas (Fig. 30–2).

The spleen now remains attached to the gastrosplenic ligament. The gastrosplenic ligament is divided just outside the gastroepiploic arcade.

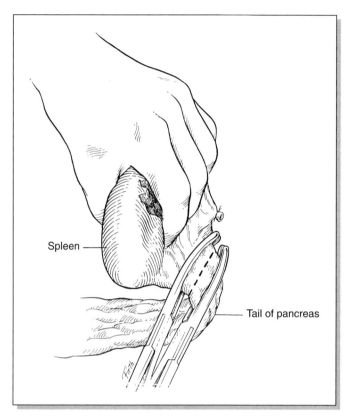

FIGURE 30–2 After complete mobilization of the spleen, the vessels at the hilum are clamped and divided, avoiding injury to the tail of the pancreas.

The short gastric vessels and the left gastroepiploic vessel are divided and ligated. To avoid injury to the greater curvature of the stomach, the vessels are ligated in continuity or, alternatively, fine Schnidt clamps can be used. The spleen is removed and the region is carefully inspected for hemostasis. The stomach and the tail of the pancreas are also inspected to exclude injury. Drains are usually not required unless an injury to the tail of the pancreas is suspected. The abdomen is irrigated, especially the left upper quadrant, to remove all debris and blood clots.

When the spleen is huge, the adhesions to the diaphragm are carefully divided. Rough mobilization will create unnecessary bleeding. Early control of the splenic artery is advisable; this artery can be identified at the superior border of the pancreas. Access to the splenic artery is achieved by dividing the lesser omentum and retracting the stomach downward or, alternatively, by dividing the gastrocolic ligament. The splenic artery is carefully isolated with a right-angle Mixter clamp and ligated with 0-0 silk.

The short gastric vessels in the gastrosplenic ligament are also divided and ligated. The splenic vessels are carefully isolated at the hilum, divided, and ligated as described earlier. Alternatively, the vessels in the hilum can be serially transected with an endovascular stapler.

CLOSURE   The midline incision is closed by approximating the linea alba with 1-0 polypropylene monofilament sutures. The left costal incision is approximated in layers with 1-0 absorbable monofilament sutures. The skin is closed with staples.

CHAPTER 31

Laparoscopic Splenectomy

EMBRYOLOGY AND ANATOMY   See Chapter 30.

Operative Procedure

PREOPERATIVE PREPARATION   This is the same as for open splenectomy.

POSITION   The patient is placed in the Lloyd-Davies position with the use of Allen stirrups, as described in Chapter 36. This allows the surgeon to stand between the legs of the patient. The patient is rolled to the right side by placement of a longitudinally oriented roll behind the left thoracoabdominal area.

ESTABLISHMENT OF PNEUMOPERITONEUM   Standard pneumoperitoneum is established through a supraumbilical approach. After this an umbilical port is placed and the camera inserted through it.

PLACEMENT OF PORTS   The four remaining ports are placed such that they form a semicircle facing the spleen: A subxiphoid retraction port is placed in the midline, a second retraction port is placed midway between the xiphoid and the umbilical port, and the third and fourth ports are placed in the left upper quadrant, one in the midaxillary line and one in the anterior axillary line.

EXPOSURE AND OPERATIVE TECHNIQUE   First, a thorough laparoscopic exploration of the abdomen is performed, with special attention directed to excluding accessory splenic tissue. To allow for improved access to the spleen, the operating table is rolled toward the right side. Initially, the splenocolic ligament is sharply divided. Any vessels that are present can be secured with the use of a harmonic scalpel or hemoclips. The splenic hilum is carefully exposed. Under direct vision the splenic vessels are carefully freed and divided using an endovascular linear stapling device (Fig. 31–1). The short gastric vessels can be addressed in a similar fashion or can be divided with the use of a harmonic scalpel. Great care is taken to avoid injury to the greater curvature of the stomach while securing the short gastric vessels. Next, the remaining splenic ligaments are divided. The spleen is captured into a large retrieval bag. If an intact spleen is to be removed, one of the abdominal incisions is extended. Alternatively, the spleen can be morselized and then removed through one of the ports. The left upper quadrant is irrigated and any blood clots aspirated. The abdominal cavity is deflated, and the port sites are inspected for bleeding.

CLOSURE   The fascial defects at the port sites are closed with figure-of-eight sutures using 0-0 absorbable sutures. The skin is approximated with subcuticular absorbable sutures and reinforced with Steri-Strips.

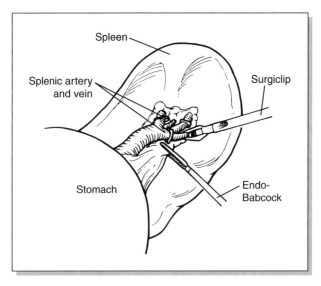

FIGURE 31–1 The hilar vessels are exposed and can be transected with an endovascular stapler.

LARGE BOWEL/ANORECTUM

CHAPTER 32

Appendectomy

EMBRYOLOGY   During the early developmental stage, the appendix is the caudal extension of the cecum and possesses the same caliber. The right wall of the cecum grows rapidly downward and begins to displace the appendix medially and closer to the ileocecal area.

ANATOMY   The appendix varies in length from 8 to 14 cm and arises from the posteromedial surface of the cecum, where all three taeniae coli meet. The position of the appendix can vary considerably among patients. It can be located in the pelvis, behind or along the lateral border of the cecum, or anterior or posterior to the distal ileum. The appendix possesses a complete peritoneal covering and has its own mesoappendix, which is attached to the mesentery of the distal ileum. Contained within the mesoappendix is the appendicular artery, which is a branch of the posterior cecal artery. Venous drainage of the appendix is via the appendicular vein, which drains into the posterior cecal vein. The nerve supply of the appendix is derived from both sympathetic and vagal fibers. Visceral pain from the appendix is conducted by the afferent sympathetic fibers that enter at the T10 spinal level.

PREOPERATIVE PREPARATION   Once a diagnosis of acute appendicitis is entertained and a decision is made to explore the patient, it is imperative to resuscitate the patient adequately with intravenous fluids. Intravenous antibiotics should be administered. In young patients, minimal investigations are required if the clinical picture is strongly suspicious for appendicitis. If a mass is palpable in the right lower quadrant, computed tomography of the abdomen and pelvis can be valuable to assess for the presence of either an appendiceal abscess or a malignant tumor arising from the cecum, appendix, or small bowel. Depending on the expertise of the radiographer, often an ultrasound can be used for visualization of the thickened appendix.

Operative Procedure

POSITION   The patient is placed in the supine position and undergoes general anesthesia with endotracheal intubation. While the patient is anesthetized and the abdominal musculature relaxed, it is advisable to carefully examine the abdomen to ascertain the presence of right lower quadrant masses. If there is any uncertainty about the diagnosis of appendicitis, especially in females, a lower midline incision can be made. Alternatively, the procedure may initially begin with diagnostic laparoscopy. If, however, the clinical suspicion for appendicitis is high, the direct approach to the appendix via the right lower quadrant is made.

INCISION   McBurney's point, located one third of the distance from the anterior superior iliac spine to the umbilicus, is identified. A transverse skin incision (Rocky-Davis incision) is made at McBurney's point (Fig. 32–1A). The skin incision should be long enough to allow the appendectomy to be performed without unnecessary excessive retraction of the anterior abdominal musculature and skin.

EXPOSURE AND OPERATIVE TECHNIQUE   The skin incision is carried through the subcutaneous tissue until the external oblique fascia is exposed. A small incision is made in the external oblique fascia along the line of its fibers. The superior and the inferior edges of this opening are grasped with curved Kelly clamps. This incision is sharply extended with slightly open Metzenbaum scissors along the direction of the fibers (Fig. 32–1B). The underlying fibers of the internal oblique muscle are identified and split with a curved Kelly clamp and retracted with Army-Navy or Richardson retractors.

Next, the transversus abdominis muscle is identified and split and the Richardson retractors adjusted to expose the peritoneum. The operator grasps the peritoneum with curved Kelly clamps, carefully verifying that intra-abdominal viscera have not been inadvertently grasped. With a no. 15 scalpel, a small incision is made in the peritoneum. Suction catheters and culture swabs should be available in case purulent fluid is encountered when the peritoneal cavity is entered. If this is the case, some fluid should be obtained for bacteriologic culture and the rest aspirated to limit any contamination of the wound edges. The edges of the peritoneum are

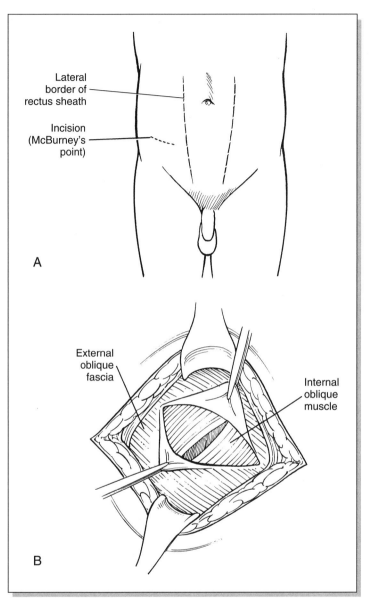

FIGURE 32–1   *A,* The transverse incision is placed at McBurney's point. *B,* The external oblique fascia is incised and the underlying muscles are split.

Illustration continued on the following page

grasped with curved Kelly clamps, and the peritoneal opening is extended with Metzenbaum scissors. If there is any difficulty gaining access to the cecum, the transversus and the internal oblique muscles may be divided with electrocautery. A medium Richardson retractor can be placed within the peritoneal cavity to elevate the anterior abdominal wall. The cecum is delivered into the wound, and the taeniae coli are followed to identify the appendix. Before the appendix is delivered, the wound edges are protected with moist laparotomy pads. If difficulty is encountered in delivering the cecum, the peritoneal lining along the lateral paracolic area may need to be divided to mobilize the cecum. Often the appendix will be found adherent to the cecum with either congenital or inflammatory adhesions, which must be divided carefully with a combination of electrocautery and Metzenbaum scissors.

As the appendix is freed, it is gently grasped with a Babcock clamp. If the mesoappendix is not thick, inflamed, and edematous, a small window is created at the base of the appendix and the mesoappendix is doubly clamped with Kelly clamps. The vessels within the mesoappendix are ligated with 2-0 silk sutures (Fig. 32–1C). If the mesoappendix is very edematous and friable, it is advisable to serially ligate the mesoappendix in continuity with 2-0 silk. The mesoappendix is divided and further suture ligated proximally with 3-0 silk. While addressing the mesoappendix, it is advisable to wrap the inflamed appendix in a gauze sponge to avoid direct contact with the wound margins and thus prevent wound infections. The base of the appendix is then gently crushed with a straight clamp. The

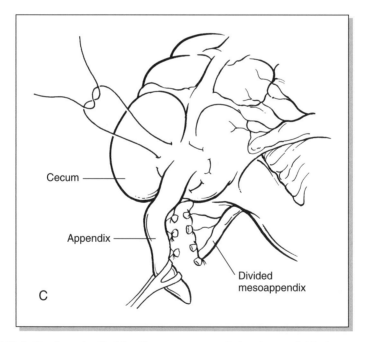

Cecum

Appendix

Divided
mesoappendix

C

FIGURE 32–1 *Continued.* *C,* After the mesoappendix has been divided, a purse-string suture using an absorbable suture can be placed to invert the base of the appendix.

base is doubly ligated with 2-0 absorbable sutures. A straight hemostat is placed on the appendix approximately 1.5 cm distal to the ligature, and the appendix is transected with a scalpel. The specimen and the contaminated instruments are removed from the operative field.

One way of managing the stump is to cleanse it with Betadine and then electrocoagulate its mucosa. Alternatively, some surgeons prefer placing a purse-string suture around the base of the appendix using 3-0 absorbable sutures and then inverting the appendiceal stump (see Fig. 32–1*C*). In cases of severe appendicitis where the base of the cecum has become inflamed and edematous and poses a risk for inadequate closure of the appendiceal stump at its base, partial cecectomy can be performed with an endo-GIA linear stapling device. The mesentery is checked for hemostasis before the cecum is returned to the abdomen. Often the gas within the lumen expands the cecum so that it may be difficult to return it to the peritoneal cavity. In this case the cecum is deflated gently by compressing it to squeeze the gas into the ascending colon.

If an acutely inflamed appendix had been found and removed, the rest of the abdomen does not need to be explored. However, if the appendix is not inflamed, the surgeon needs to exclude other pathologic processes that can present with right lower quadrant pain. The cecum should be palpated for the presence of any malignant masses. The terminal ileum should be examined for evidence of Crohn's disease, acute ileitis, tuberculous or actinomycotic ileitis, or a Meckel's diverticulum. In female patients the uterus, fallopian tubes, and ovaries must be palpated and examined. If further exposure of the pelvis is required, the rectus sheath and muscle may be divided. If purulent fluid or abscess is encountered, the right lower quadrant and the pelvic cavity are irrigated with sterile saline.

CLOSURE The peritoneum is grasped with curved Kelly clamps and approximated with 3-0 continuous absorbable sutures. The transversus and internal oblique muscle layers are irrigated and loosely approximated with 2-0 absorbable sutures. The external oblique fascia is repaired with continuous 0-0 absorbable sutures. The subcutaneous tissue is irrigated, and the skin is approximated with staples. If there had been excessive contamination of the wound, it should be left open and the subcutaneous tissue packed with saline-soaked gauze. A delayed primary closure can be performed by day 3 to 4.

CHAPTER 33

Laparoscopic Appendectomy

EMBRYOLOGY AND ANATOMY　See Chapter 32.

PREOPERATIVE PREPARATION　This is the same as in open appendectomy (Chapter 32).

Operative Procedure

ESTABLISHMENT OF PNEUMOPERITONEUM　Intra-abdominal CO_2 insufflation is established in the usual fashion through the primary periumbilical port. The patient is placed in the Trendelenburg position to improve visualization of the pelvis and lower abdomen. A standard diagnostic laparoscopic examination of the abdominal cavity is performed.

PLACEMENT OF PORTS　Two ports are placed, a 10-mm port in the suprapubic area and a 5-mm port in the left lower quadrant. Both are directed toward the appendix.

EXPOSURE AND OPERATIVE TECHNIQUE　With a two-handed technique, the surgeon first exposes the appendix with use of an atraumatic forceps. Once located, the tip of the appendix is grasped with an atraumatic forceps and lifted upward toward the abdominal wall. The mesoappendix is dissected close to the base of the appendix with a curved forceps. The mesoappendix is divided using an endovascular linear stapler (Fig. 33–1). The base of the appendix is carefully freed of any surrounding adipose tissue and transected at its base using an endo-GIA stapler. The resected appendix is placed within a specimen retrieval bag and removed. The right lower quadrant is irrigated with saline to remove any contaminated material. If any difficulty is encountered during dissection, the procedure should be converted to an open appendectomy.

CLOSURE   The fascial defects are closed with figure-of-eight sutures using 0-0 absorbable sutures and the skin is closed with subcuticular absorbable sutures.

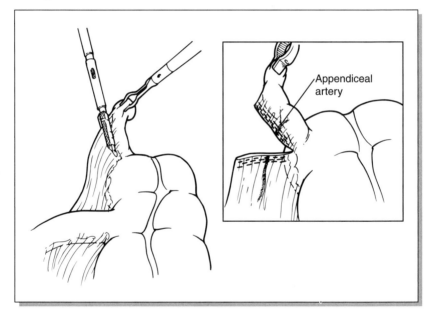

FIGURE 33–1   The mesoappendix is dissected close to the base of the appendix and then divided with an endovascular stapler.

CHAPTER 34

Colon Resection

EMBRYOLOGY   The cecum, ascending colon, and proximal third of the transverse colon are derived from the midgut. The rest of the large bowel, rectum, and upper part of the anal canal develops from the hindgut. The cecal swelling is the last part of the midgut to reenter the abdominal cavity. The cecal bud is originally present in the right upper quadrant, where it forms the cecum and the appendix and subsequently descends into the right iliac fossa, thereby forming the ascending colon and the hepatic flexure. Once the colon has reached its definitive position, the mesenteries of the ascending and descending colons fuse with the posterior abdominal wall, thus rendering them retroperitoneal structures. The transverse colon and the sigmoid colon retain their mesentery.

ANATOMY   The large intestine extends from the ileocecal junction to the anal orifice and measures approximately 103 cm long. It can be distinguished from the small bowel by the following features: (1) presence of teniae, which are three bands of longitudinal muscle; (2) the appendices epiploicae, which are fatty appendages projecting from the serosal surface of the bowel; and (3) the haustra, which are sacculations caused by the longitudinal muscle's being shorter than the rest of the bowel wall. The components of large intestine include the cecum, appendix, ascending colon, transverse colon, descending colon, sigmoid colon, rectum, and anal canal. The appendix is considered in Chapter 32, and the rectum and anal canal are considered in Chapter 36.

Cecum The cecum is a dilated pouch measuring about 6 to 8 cm, below the level of the ileocecal valve. It is situated in the right lower quadrant lying on the iliacus and psoas muscles. It is completely invested with peritoneum, which allows it to be mobile. The three teniae of the cecum converge on the posteromedial aspect at the base of the appendix. The tip of the appendix is often lying in the pelvis but can also be found behind the cecum (retrocecal fossa). The ileocecal valve is an oval opening that is present on the medial aspect of the cecum. The circular muscle of the distal ileum acts as the sphincter. The arterial blood supply of the cecum is derived from anterior and posterior cecal arteries, which are branches of the ileocolic artery. The venous drainage corresponds to the arterial supply and drains into the superior mesenteric vein. The lymphatic drainage is via nodes that follow the vessels.

Ascending Colon The ascending colon (15 to 20 cm long) extends upward from the cecum and turns sharply to the left to form the hepatic flexure and then becomes continuous with the transverse colon. The peritoneum lines the anterior and lateral surfaces of the ascending colon, whereas the posterior surface lies against the posterior abdominal wall. Lateral to the ascending colon is the paracolic gutter, which leads to the subphrenic space superiorly. Posteriorly it lies on the iliacus, quadratus lumborum, and lower pole of the right kidney. It receives its arterial blood supply from the ileocolic and the right colic branches of the superior mesenteric artery. The veins correspond to the arteries and drain into the superior mesenteric vein. Lymphatic drainage is into nodes that lie along the above-named blood vessels.

Transverse Colon The transverse colon measures approximately 50 cm long and extends upward from the hepatic flexure to the left to form the splenic flexure, which is suspended from the diaphragm by the phrenicocolic ligament. It is attached by the transverse mesocolon to the anterior border of the pancreas on the posterior abdominal wall. The anterior leaf of the transverse mesocolon adheres to the greater omentum. Posteriorly the colon is related to the second part of duodenum, head of the pancreas, loops of small bowel, and left kidney. Owing to the dual embryologic origin, the proximal two thirds of the transverse colon receives its blood supply from the middle colic artery, which runs within the transverse mesocolon and is the second branch of the superior mesenteric artery. The left colic artery, a branch of the inferior mesenteric artery, supplies the distal one third of the transverse colon. The veins correspond to the arteries and drain into the superior and inferior mesenteric veins. The lymphatic drainage follows the colic blood supply.

Descending Colon This segment of the colon is the narrowest and measures approximately 30 cm. It extends downward in the left lumbar region from the splenic flexure to the pelvic brim, where it continues as the sigmoid colon. Similar to the ascending colon, the peritoneum covers the anterolateral wall and forms the left paracolic gutter. Thus, the posterior surface of the descending colon is a retroperitoneal structure. Posterior relations include the lower pole of the left kidney, diaphragm, quadratus lumborum, iliacus, and psoas muscles. The arterial blood supply is derived from the left colic branch of the inferior mesenteric artery. The vein corresponds to the artery and drains into the inferior mesenteric vein. The lymphatic drainage follows the colic blood vessels.

Sigmoid Colon   This segment of the colon measures approximately 40 cm and extends from the pelvic brim to the third sacral vertebra. It is suspended by a V-shaped sigmoid mesocolon, the apex of which is situated over the left ureter where it crosses the pelvic brim. The left limb of the V is attached along the medial aspect of the external iliac artery, and the right limb runs from the bifurcation of the left common iliac artery downward to the third sacral vertebra. The arterial blood supply of the sigmoid colon is derived from sigmoid branches of the inferior mesenteric artery, and the venous drainage is into the inferior mesenteric vein. Lymph drainage is into nodes along the inferior left colic artery and subsequently to the inferior mesenteric nodes.

PREOPERATIVE PREPARATION   In addition to assessing the cardiovascular, pulmonary, and renal function of the patient and obtaining basic laboratory studies, special studies such as barium enema are reviewed preoperatively. If the patient has a colon carcinoma, a preoperative colonoscopy is required to evaluate the colon for the presence of synchronous malignant lesions and/or polyps. Staging investigations include chest radiograph, liver function tests, serum carcinoembryonic antigen, and computed tomography of the abdomen and pelvis. The colon lesion should have undergone biopsy and the pathology reviewed.

Standard preoperative bowel preparation can be achieved either with 4 L of GoLYTELY (polyethylene glycol–electrolyte) solution or magnesium citrate. Neomycin and erythromycin in three separate doses, 1 g each at 1:00 PM, 2:00 PM, and 11:00 PM, are administered orally. Perioperatively the patient is given a prophylactic antibiotic dose such as cefoxitin 2 g intravenously and metronidazole 500 mg intravenously, as well as 5000 units of heparin subcutaneously.

Operative Procedure

The various types of standard colon resections performed and the extent of large bowel removed are indicated in Figure 34–1. In this chapter right, left, and sigmoid colectomy are described.

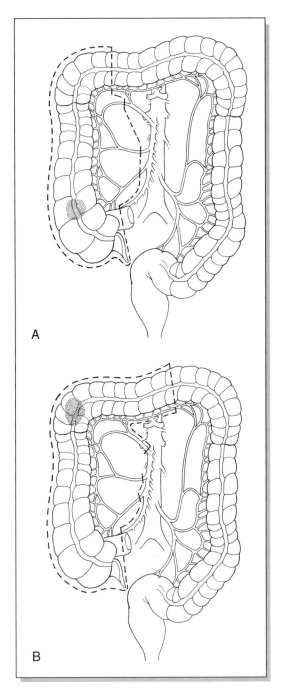

FIGURE 34–1 The various types of colon resections performed; dashed lines indicate the extent of large bowel removed. *A*, Right hemicolectomy; *B*, extended right colectomy.

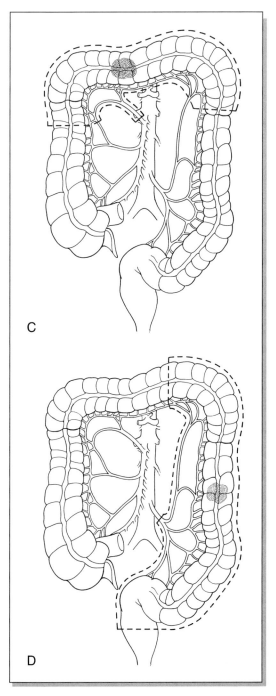

FIGURE 34–1 *Continued.* *C*, Transverse colectomy; *D*, left colectomy.
Illustration continued on the following page

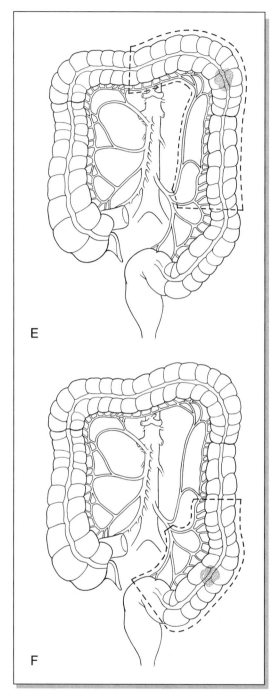

FIGURE 34–1 *Continued.* *E,* Extended left colectomy; *F,* sigmoid colectomy.

Right Hemicolectomy

POSITION   The patient is placed in the supine position, and a nasogastric tube and Foley catheters are inserted. Sequential pneumatic compression devices are placed to prevent deep venous thrombosis.

INCISION   A midline incision is the incision of choice because it allows a thorough exploration and intraoperative staging of the patient's disease. Some surgeons prefer a transverse incision placed midway between the costal margin and the iliac crest and extending across the midline just below the umbilicus. A thorough exploration is performed, including assessment for peritoneal implants and bimanual palpation of the liver to exclude metastases. The small bowel is packed away on the left side of the abdomen. A self-retaining retractor system is arranged for optimal exposure.

EXPOSURE AND OPERATIVE TECHNIQUE   The assistant grasps the right colon with moist gauze and retracts it medially. Dissection for the entire procedure can be performed with either Metzenbaum scissors or electrocautery. The avascular line of Toldt along the right paracolic gutter is incised from the cecum to the hepatic flexure. This allows the right colon to be lifted and rotated medially. Incising the additional lateral peritoneal coverings further mobilizes the colon. The dissection is extended across the ileocolic junction and completed by mobilization of the terminal ileum. Next, the right ureter is identified before any deeper dissection is performed. The ureter is usually located at the bifurcation of the right common iliac artery; if it is not found, meticulous dissection beneath the lateral and medial peritoneal folds will usually locate it. Once the ureter is identified, it should be pushed gently away from the operative specimen toward the posterior abdominal wall. Often it is helpful to place a vessel loop around it for identification and to maintain it continuously in the surgeon's visual field, while proceeding with the remainder of the dissection.

Mobilization of the right colon is continued by dividing the thin adventitial layers. This dissection is performed with a meticulous combination of blunt and sharp dissection. The following vital structures then come into view: the right kidney, ureter, gonadal vessels, and duodenum. The kidney, ureter, and gonadal vessels are carefully dissected and preserved. Next, the second portion of the duodenum is carefully separated from the specimen.

With moist gauze, the operator retracts the hepatic flexure caudally and mobilizes it by dividing the peritoneum in the hepatorenal fossa. This dissection is continued medially by dividing the right margin of the gastrocolic ligament between large clamps and ligating it with 2-0 silk sutures. This part of the mobilization should be done with care, because the omentum adheres to the anterior leaf of the transverse mesocolon, and the middle colic vessels with the mesocolon can be inadvertently injured.

Once mobilization has been accomplished, the vascular arcade of the specimen is visualized by transillumination, and the line of transection of the distal ileum and the transverse colon is determined. For neoplasms close to the ileocecal junction, about 10 to 15 cm of the terminal ileum must be resected. For tumors adjacent to the hepatic flexure, approximately 8 to 10 cm of ileum must be removed. At the determined site of ileal transection, a small opening is made in the mesentery and the ileum is transected with a GIA-60 stapler. The GIA-60 stapler is reloaded, and the transverse colon is transected in a similar fashion. The peritoneal covering on the medial aspect of the mesentery is scored with electrocautery. The vessels within the ileal mesentery are serially clamped, divided, and ligated with 2-0 or 3-0 silk sutures. Avascular parts of the mesentery can be divided with electrocautery. The ileocolic, right colic, and right branch of the middle colic artery are identified and individually clamped, divided, and serially ligated with 2-0 silk sutures. It is often preferable to place transfixion suture ligatures on the proximal end of these named vessels with 3-0 silk sutures. The specimen is removed and inspected on the back table.

The adequacy of the blood supply at the ends of the ileum and transverse colon is determined. The end of the transverse colon is cleared of pericolic adipose tissue in preparation for anastomosis. The ileocolic anastomosis can be either hand sewn or stapled end to end or end to side. Atraumatic Doyen or Glanzmann bowel clamps are placed on the ileum and the transverse colon to prevent spillage of bowel contents. The area of the anastomosis is separated from the rest of the abdominal cavity with laparotomy pads as a precautionary measure to contain any spillage. For a hand-sewn anastomosis, first the posterior seromuscular layer of interrupted 3-0 silk Lembert sutures is placed. The staple line of both the ileum and the transverse colon is excised, and because there is usually a disparity in the diameter of the two ends, a 1- to 2-cm Cheadle incision is made on the antimesenteric border of the ileum. Next, an inner layer of continuous 4-0 absorbable sutures is placed and converted to Connell sutures anteriorly. Placing the anterior seromuscular layer with interrupted 3-0 silk Lembert sutures completes the anastomosis. A similar two-layer technique can be used for an end-to-side anastomosis.

Alternatively, a stapled functional end-to-end anastomosis can be constructed. First, the two cut ends of the ileum and the colon are aligned by placing a 2-0 silk seromuscular stay suture. To facilitate construction of the anastomosis, a similar stay suture is placed about 6 to 7 cm from these cut ends. The antimesenteric corner of the staple line on the ileum and the transverse colon is excised to create a small opening for insertion of the stapling device. One fork of the GIA-60 instrument is inserted into each bowel lumen. The instrument is closed, and the mesentery is inspected to ensure that it is not caught within the instrument. The stapling device is fired, resulting in a 4- to 5-cm side-to-side anastomosis. The end of the bowel is grasped with Allis clamps and the staple line inspected for hemostasis and any defects. The same Allis clamps are used to approximate the common opening, which is closed with a TA-55 stapling device or hand sewn with a double layer of sutures. Finally, the mesenteric defect is closed with continuous 3-0 absorbable sutures, with particular attention to avoiding injuring to any vessels lying in the free margin of the mesentery, because this may compromise the blood supply of the anastomosis. Once the anastomosis is complete, the instruments and laparotomy pads used up to this point are discarded. The surgical team changes gloves and prepares to close the abdomen.

CLOSURE   The abdominal cavity is finally checked for hemostasis and irrigated with warm saline solution. The greater omentum may be used to cover the anastomosis. The linea alba is approximated with continuous 1-0 monofilament nonabsorbable sutures. The subcutaneous tissue is irrigated with saline solution, hemostasis is secured, and the skin is closed with staples. If contamination has occurred, it is best to pack the subcutaneous tissue with saline-moistened gauze packs and leave the skin incision open.

Left Hemicolectomy

POSITION   The patient is usually placed in the supine position. However, if the dissection may involve removal of part of the rectum and access to the anal canal may be needed, the patient should be placed in the Lloyd-Davies position. In this position the patient's buttocks are elevated with a towel roll and the legs are placed in stirrups, which allows the hips to be flexed and abducted and the knees flexed. A Foley catheter and a nasogastric tube are inserted, and perioperative prophylactic antibiotics are given. The patient's abdomen is prepped and draped from the nipple down to the thighs. Sequential pneumatic compression devices are applied, or a prophylactic dose of subcutaneous heparin is administered.

INCISION   The standard incision is usually the midline, usually from the level of the pubis to above the umbilicus to a varying length. If the procedure is for colonic malignancy, the incision extends from the xiphoid to the pubis to allow adequate staging of the patient.

EXPOSURE AND OPERATIVE TECHNIQUE   Once the abdomen is entered in the usual fashion, a thorough exploration is performed to exclude any unsuspected intra-abdominal pathology. In the case of malignancy, any evidence of metastatic disease should be determined. The patient is placed in a reverse Trendelenburg position, and the small bowel is packed to the right side to improve exposure. Excessive retraction on the small bowel should be avoided because it may cause tears in the mesentery.

The descending colon is drawn medially, and the line of Toldt in the paracolic gutter is sharply incised and extended downward to the sigmoid colon to the level of the rectosigmoid junction. The sigmoid colon is next grasped and lifted to demonstrate the V-shaped mesocolon. The peritoneum at the apex of the mesocolon is incised to allow identification of the left ureter as it crosses the common iliac vessels. Gently compressing the ureter with a DeBakey forceps to observe its peristalsis of the ureter is a useful maneuver. The ureter is encircled with a vessel loop and displaced away from the operative field to preserve its integrity. Lateral to the ureter are the gonadal vessels. With these structures in view, the lateral peritoneal fold is incised superiorly toward the splenic flexure. The operator further mobilizes the left colon away from the posterior abdominal wall by dividing the areolar tissue with electrocautery. The operator gently retracts the splenic flexure downward with a laparotomy pad while the assistant firmly retracts the left costal margin.

The peritoneal covering around the splenic flexure is dissected using a right-angle Mixter clamp and divided with electrocautery. Next, the underlying splenocolic ligament and the more medially located pancreaticocolic ligaments are divided, allowing further mobilization of the splenic flexure. The distal transverse colon is separated from the stomach by serially dividing and ligating the greater omentum outside the gastroepiploic arcade. The approximate point of division of the transverse colon is selected, and an opening is made in the adjacent mesentery. The bowel is transected with a linear stapling device. The peritoneum on the medial aspect of the mesentery is scored, and the vessels are serially clamped, divided, and ligated individually with 2-0 silk ligatures.

The dissection proceeds toward the inferior mesenteric artery, which is identified, carefully isolated, ligated in continuity with 0-0 silk sutures, and divided. The proximal end is further secured by placing a 2-0 transfixion silk suture. Dissection is continued distally in the mesentery where the sigmoidal arteries are divided. The rectosigmoid junction and the upper rectum now remain to be mobilized. The dissected bowel is retracted anteriorly, and the adjacent peritoneal covering on each side is extended toward the pelvis. The loose areolar tissue in the presacral space is dissected sharply with electrocautery to the level of the sacral promontory, ensuring at least a 5-cm distal margin from the tumor. At the level of the rectosigmoid junction, the bowel is transected with either a GIA-60 or a TA-55 stapler, depending on the access to the area. The ends of the bowel are inspected, and the pericolonic adipose tissue is removed for at least 1 cm in preparation for the anastomosis.

The greater omentum should be dissected along the avascular plane to mobilize the transverse colon and allow it to reach the sigmoid colon for a tension-free anastomosis. After ensuring that there is no twisting of the mesentery, the operator aligns the bowel ends. Atraumatic bowel clamps are placed to prevent spillage, and the rest of the abdomen is isolated with laparotomy pads.

A two-layer anastomosis can be constructed with an inner layer of continuous sutures encompassing all layers using 3-0 absorbable sutures followed by an outer seromuscular layer of interrupted 3-0 silk Lembert sutures. To perform a stapled anastomosis, the staple line from the distal colon is excised and the edges are grasped with three Allis clamps. The diameter of the EEA instrument to be used is determined using the EEA sizers. Next, a purse-string suture using 3-0 polypropylene is placed around the distal colon either manually or with the purse-string instrument. The anvil is introduced into the distal colon, and the purse-string suture is tied down. Approximately 5 cm from the edge of the proximal colon, a longitudinal colotomy is made. The EEA instrument is placed into the colon and slowly opened to advance the rod through the middle of the staple line. The EEA shaft is engaged to the anvil, the instrument is closed, and the staples are fired. The colotomy is closed transversely with a TA-55 stapler. The bowel clamps are removed and the abdomen copiously irrigated with saline.

CLOSURE   The midline incision is closed in a standard fashion by approximating the linea alba with continuous 1-0 polypropylene monofilament sutures.

Sigmoid Colectomy

POSITION   The patient is placed in the supine position. However, if the dissection may involve removal of part of the rectum and access to the anal canal may be needed, the patient should be placed in the Lloyd-Davies position. A Foley and a nasogastric tube are inserted. Perioperative prophylactic antibiotics are administered. The patient's abdomen is prepped and draped from the nipple down to the thighs.

INCISION   The lower midline incision is standard, usually from the level of the pubis to above the umbilicus to a varying length. If the procedure is performed for colonic malignancy, the incision extends from the xiphoid to the pubis to allow accurate staging of the cancer.

EXPOSURE AND OPERATIVE TECHNIQUE   Once the abdomen is entered in the usual fashion, a thorough exploration is performed to exclude any unsuspected intra-abdominal pathology. In the case of malignancy, metastatic disease should be sought and identified. The patient is placed in a reverse Trendelenburg position, and the small bowel is packed to the right side to improve exposure. Excessive retraction on the small bowel is avoided because it may cause tears in the mesentery. The sigmoid colon is lifted to visualize the V-shaped mesentery. Starting at the apex of the mesentery, the peritoneal lining is scored on both sides with electrocautery. The left ureter should be located at the level of the sigmoid fossa (i.e., apex of the sigmoid mesocolon). Sigmoid resection is started by making a small opening on the mesenteric aspect of the junction between the descending colon and the sigmoid colon. Here, the large bowel is transected with a linear GIA-60 stapler.

The sigmoid vessels within the mesentery are identified, serially clamped, divided, and ligated with 2-0 silk sutures. As the apex of the sigmoid vessels is approached, the previously identified ureter should be kept in full view before clamping any vessels. If the sigmoid resection is for diverticular disease, a wide resection of the mesentery is not needed. Before division and ligation of the vessels along the inferior limb of the sigmoid mesocolon, the right ureter should be identified and preserved. After these vessels have been secured, the rectosigmoid junction is divided with a linear GIA-60 stapler (Fig. 34–2A).

The descending colon and, if necessary, the splenic flexure are now mobilized. If the sigmoid resection is being performed for acute complicated diverticulitis or malignant tumor, a Hartmann's procedure is performed. This involves bringing the descending colon out as an end-colostomy and leaving the rectal stump either closed or, rarely, brought to the anterior abdominal wall as a mucous fistula.

For an elective case, an end-to-end colonic hand-sewn or stapled anastomosis is constructed. For a hand-sewn anastomosis, either a single- or a two-layer technique can be used. First, a noncrushing Glanzmann bowel clamp is placed on the descending colon and the rectum to avoid any spillage. The area of anastomosis is isolated from the rest of the abdomen with laparotomy pads. For a single-layer anastomosis, multiple 2-0 silk sutures encompassing all the layers are placed (Fig. 34–2B). Once all the sutures are placed, the descending colon is parachuted down toward the rectum and the sutures are tied down securely. A two-layered anastomosis is begun with an outer posterior layer of interrupted Lembert sutures using 3-0 silk. Next, the inner layer encompassing all layers of the bowel is begun with continuous 3-0 absorbable sutures, converting the anterior layer to Connell sutures. Placing the anterior layer of interrupted seromuscular 3-0 silk Lembert sutures completes the anastomosis.

For a stapled anastomosis, a purse-string suture using 3-0 monofilament nonabsorbable sutures is placed manually or with a purse-string instrument along the transected rectal stump. The diameter of the rectum

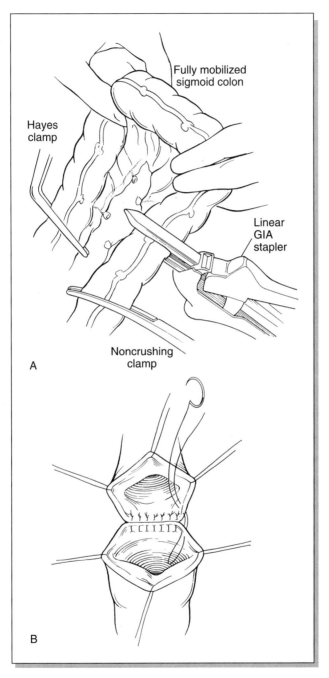

FIGURE 34–2 *A*, After division of the vessels in the mesocolon, soft clamps are placed across the bowel, which is then divided with a linear GIA stapler. *B*, Bowel anastomosis is being performed with a hand-sewn technique.

is determined using the EEA sizers. The appropriately sized EEA instrument is introduced in the descending colon through a longitudinal colotomy performed 3 to 4 cm proximal to the anastomotic site and along the steniae. The EEA instrument is opened and the spike is brought out along the side of the stapled end. The anvil is placed in the rectal stump, and the purse-string suture is secured. The anvil is engaged, the instrument is closed, and the staples are fired. The anastomosis is inspected for hemostasis, after the EEA instrument has been carefully removed. The colotomy is closed transversely either manually or with the TA-55 stapler.

CLOSURE   Midline abdominal incision is closed in the usual fashion.

CHAPTER 35

Subtotal Colectomy/ Panproctocolectomy and J-Pouch Reconstruction

ANATOMY AND EMBRYOLOGY See Chapter 34.

PREOPERATIVE PREPARATION Preparation of the patient is similar to that outlined in Chapter 34. It is advisable to have the patient seen by an enterostomal therapist to mark the site of a possible diverting ileostomy.

Operative Procedure

POSITION The patient is placed in a modified Lloyd-Davies position. The patient undergoes general anesthesia with an endotracheal intubation; a nasogastric tube and a Foley catheter are placed. Sequential compression devices are placed on the lower extremities, or, alternatively, 5000 IU of heparin can be administered subcutaneously for deep vein thrombosis prophylaxis. Perioperative antibiotics are administered. The patient is prepped and draped in the usual sterile fashion.

INCISION A midline incision that is scattered down through the subcutaneous tissue to the linea alba is made. The linea alba is then incised, and the peritoneal cavity is entered.

EXPOSURE AND OPERATIVE TECHNIQUE   A thorough exploration of the abdomen is performed. A total colectomy is begun by first dividing the peritoneal attachments of the terminal ileum and the right colon along the avascular line of Toldt. This incision is carried upward and around the hepatic flexure. If the resection is being performed for a malignant process, the greater omentum is resected along with the specimen, and in this case the transverse colon is separated from the stomach by division of the gastrocolic ligament. This ligament can be divided with a harmonic scalpel; alternatively, the vessels within the ligament are serially clamped, divided, and ligated with 2-0 silk sutures. If the resection of the colon is being performed for a benign process, the greater omentum is preserved by detaching it from the transverse colon. This mobilization is continued toward the splenic flexure, where the splenocolic ligament is carefully divided with electrocautery. Particular attention is taken to avoid injury to the splenic capsule. Next, the lateral peritoneal attachments of the descending colon are incised down to the level of the sacral promontory. On the right side, the duodenum and the ureter are identified and preserved. In a similar fashion, on the left side, the left ureter is also identified and gently retracted posteriorly to avoid injury.

After total mobilization of the abdominal colon (Fig. 35–1), the arcades of the terminal ileum are serially clamped, divided, and ligated with 2-0 silk sutures. Next, the right colic, middle colic, left colic, and sigmoidal vessels are sequentially divided between clamps and ligated with 0-0 silk sutures. The major vessels are further secured with 2-0 silk transfixion sutures. The distal ileum is divided with a GIA-60 linear stapler. If the rectum is to be spared, the bowel is transected at the rectosigmoid junction with a TA-55 stapler.

A double-stapled side-to-end ileorectal anastomosis can be constructed with a circular EEA stapler. For this the anus is gently dilated. Then the circular stapler, without the anvil, is placed into the rectum through the anus. The trocar is used to penetrate just anterior to the staple line. A Doyen bowel clamp is placed across the distal ileum. An enterotomy is made on the antimesenteric border of the terminal ileum. A purse-string suture using a 3-0 monofilament nonabsorbable suture is placed around the enterotomy. The anvil is gently passed into the small bowel, and the purse-string is tied securely. The anvil is engaged to the stapling device, which is closed and fired.

If panproctocolectomy is to be performed, the rectum is mobilized within the pelvic cavity as described in Chapter 36. At the level of the dentate line, the rectum is transected using a TA-55 reticulating stapling device.

If a J-pouch anal anastomosis is to be constructed, the ileocolic artery is divided without compromising the blood supply of the terminal ileum. To create the J-pouch, a 12-cm segment is doubled on itself to create a 6-cm-long pouch (Fig. 35–2A). The two limbs of the bowel are aligned by 3-0 silk

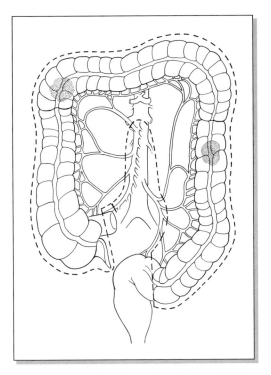

FIGURE 35–1 Extent of resection of the large bowel for subtotal colectomy (dashed lines).

stay sutures. Soft Doyen bowel clamps are placed across the small intestine. An enterotomy is made at the apex of the pouch, which is the antimesenteric surface of the small bowel (see Fig. 35–2A). The two limbs of the GIA linear stapler are inserted through the enterotomy at the apex of the J-pouch (Fig. 35–2B). After it has been ensured that the mesentery is not caught within the jaws, the stapler is closed and fired to create a side-to-side anastomosis. The stapler is removed and reloaded, because a second and often a third firing are necessary to complete the J-pouch construction. Next, a purse-string suture is placed around the enterotomy using a 3-0 monofilament non-absorbable suture (Fig. 35–2C). The anvil of the circular EEA stapling device is passed through the enterotomy, and the purse-string suture is tied down. The circular stapling device is passed through the dilated anus into the anorectal stump. The trocar is advanced through the transverse staple line and engaged with the anvil in the J-pouch. The stapler is closed and fired.

If a hand-sewn ileoanal anastomosis is to be constructed, a retractor is arranged around the anus to assist in defacement of the anal margin. The distal end of the J-pouch is gently pulled through the anal canal by the surgeon. The enterotomy of the J-pouch is anchored to the dentate line

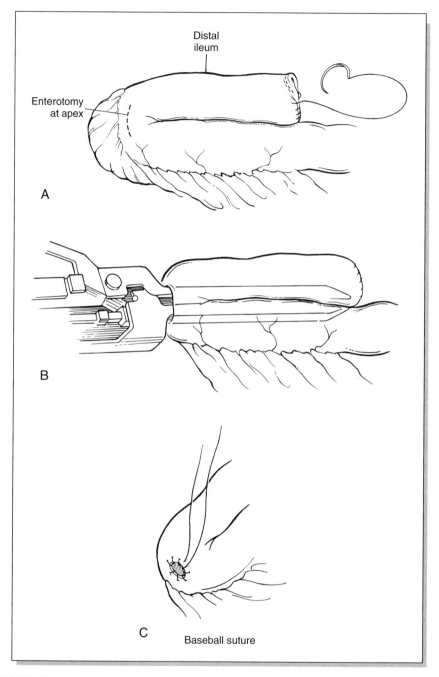

FIGURE 35–2 *A,* The terminal ileum is folded and an enterotomy is made at the apex of the J-pouch. *B,* Creation of the side-to-side anastomosis with a GIA stapler. *C,* Placement of a purse-string suture around the enterotomy.

with 3-0 absorbable sutures placed at the four corners. Additionally, two or three sutures are placed between these anchoring sutures. Once the retractor is removed, the anal canal will retract and reduce the tension on the anastomosis. Such a low ileoanal anastomosis often may need to be protected with a diverting ileostomy.

CLOSURE   The midline incision is closed in the usual fashion by approximating the linea alba with 1-0 monofilament nonabsorbable sutures. The skin is approximated with staples. If an ileostomy is being performed, it should be matured in the usual fashion at this time after covering the wound.

CHAPTER 36

Rectal Resection

EMBRYOLOGY   The rectum and the proximal part of the anal canal (i.e., to the level of the pectinate line) are derived from the hindgut. The distal segment of the anal canal develops from the proctoderm. The expanded lower part of the hindgut, known as the cloaca, is in direct contact with the surface ectoderm, the cloacal membrane. The allantois, which is a diverticulum of the yolk sac, opens on the ventral aspect of the cloaca. A sheet of mesenchymal tissue known as the urorectal septum grows caudally between the allantois and the cloaca and partitions the cloaca into an anterior portion, the primitive urogenital sinus, and a posterior part, the anorectal canal. The urorectal septum continues to grow caudally and fuses with the cloacal membrane, and this area of fusion represents the perineal body in adults. This fusion creates the anterior urogenital membrane and the posterior anorectal membrane. The blood supply of the anus can be explained by the different embryologic origins of its superior and inferior segments. The upper two thirds of the anal canal is derived from the endoderm and is therefore supplied by the artery of the hindgut, the inferior mesenteric artery, whereas the distal third of the anus is ectodermal in origin and is supplied by branches of the internal iliac artery.

ANATOMY   The rectum extends from the sigmoid colon to the anal canal. It measures approximately 12 to 13 cm and begins in front of the first sacral vertebra and follows the hollow of the sacrum to end at the level of the tip of the coccyx. When viewed in the coronal view, the rectum deviates initially to the left and then returns to the midline. In the sagittal plane the rectum can be seen following the concavity of the sacrum and inferiorly widens to form the rectal ampulla and then passes downward and posteriorly to join the anal canal. The rectum does not have a mesentery, but the peritoneum covers the lateral and anterior surfaces of the upper third of the rectum; only the anterior surface of the middle third and the lower third has no peritoneal covering.

Several fasciae of the rectum are of surgical importance. The visceral pelvic fascia (also known as rectal fascia propria) surrounds the mesorectum posteriorly. This fascial envelope encloses fat, blood vessels, nerves, and lymphatics of the rectum. Between the rectal fascia propria and the parietal (presacral) fascia is loose areolar tissue that is the plane of dissection when performing total mesorectal excision. The parietal fascia, which lines the pelvic walls, is known as the presacral fascia in the region of the sacrum. The presacral fascia is tightly adherent to concavity of the sacral periosteum, especially in the midline and around the anterior sacral foramina. The presacral fascia protects the presacral veins and the hypogastric plexus lying beneath it. The fascia of Waldeyer is a more membranous portion of the pelvic fascia that extends from the sacrum to the rectal ampulla. Just above the pelvic floor there is condensation of areolar tissue around the middle rectal vessels known as the lateral ligament of the rectum. Anteriorly, the Denonvilliers' fascia is adherent to the fascia propria of the rectum.

The blood supply of the rectum is from

- The superior rectal artery, which is a terminal branch of the inferior mesenteric artery
- The middle rectal artery, which is a branch of the internal iliac artery
- The inferior rectal artery, which is a branch of the internal pudendal artery

The venous drainage of the rectum follows that of the arteries, with the superior rectal vein draining into the portal circulation, whereas the middle and inferior rectal veins drain into the systemic circulation. The free communications between the rectal veins form an important portal-systemic anastomosis. The lymphatic drainage of the rectum is via lymphatics that travel along with the superior, middle, and inferior rectal arteries.

LOW ANTERIOR RESECTION

PREOPERATIVE PREPARATION   See Chapter 34 for details of preoperative preparation.

A careful rectal examination is necessary to evaluate the tumor with regard to the size, distance from the anal verge, percent of circumference involved, mobility, and presence of ulceration. Histologic diagnosis of the rectal mass should be obtained. The entire large bowel must be examined with colonoscopy to exclude the presence of synchronous malignancy and/or polyps. Endoscopic ultrasound is a valuable tool to establish the depth of tumor penetration into the rectal wall and also the presence of any enlarged perirectal lymph nodes. Preoperative staging work-up should also include liver function tests, carcinoembryonic level, chest radiograph, and computed tomography of the abdomen and pelvis.

Patients should undergo a standard bowel preparation and preoperative counseling regarding stoma care. The site for potential colostomy should be marked on the day of the surgery.

Operative Procedure

POSITION   The patient is placed in the Lloyd-Davies position, and a Foley catheter and nasogastric tube are placed. If a difficult pelvic dissection is contemplated, insertion of ureteral stents should be considered. Sequential pneumatic compression devices and/or subcutaneous heparin should be administered.

INCISION   A long midline incision is made extending from the xiphoid to the pubis.

EXPOSURE AND OPERATIVE TECHNIQUE   The abdomen is explored to exclude peritoneal dissemination and the presence of hepatic metastasis. The tumor mobility in the pelvis is assessed next. Apparent fixation to the pelvic structures may not preclude resection, because inflammatory or fibrotic reaction may account for this, particularly in cases where preoperative radiation or concurrent chemoradiation has been administered. The patient is placed in a slight Trendelenburg position, and a self-retaining retractor system is arranged to provide adequate exposure. The small bowel is carefully retracted superiorly to the right and packed with moist laparotomy pads.

The left colon is mobilized by sharp division of the avascular plane along the line of Toldt. The left ureter is identified as it crosses the pelvic brim over the left common iliac artery. A vessel loop can be placed around the ureter to allow for continuous visualization and displacement away from the operative field. An incision is made at the base of the V-shaped sigmoid mesentery on the right side, and the peritoneal incision is extended distally to the right side of the rectum. The same incision is extended superiorly to expose the origin of the inferior mesenteric artery. This vessel is carefully isolated and divided just distal to the origin of the left colic artery. The inferior mesenteric artery is ligated with 0-0 silk sutures and further reinforced with a 2-0 silk transfixion suture ligature. The peritoneal covering over the sigmoid mesocolon is scored with electrocautery, and the mesenteric vessels are divided and ligated with 2-0 silk sutures. The distal descending colon is divided with a GIA-60 stapling device. While upward and forward traction on the sigmoid colon is applied, the superior hemorrhoidal vessels are isolated, divided, and ligated. This maneuver allows entrance into the presacral space at the sacral promontory. The peritoneum on each side of the rectum is divided just medial to the ureters and extended to meet anteriorly to gain access to the seminal vesicles in males or the rectovaginal septum in females.

The plane of dissection within the pelvis is indicated in Figure 36–1. The posterior pelvic dissection is performed sharply with electrocautery to

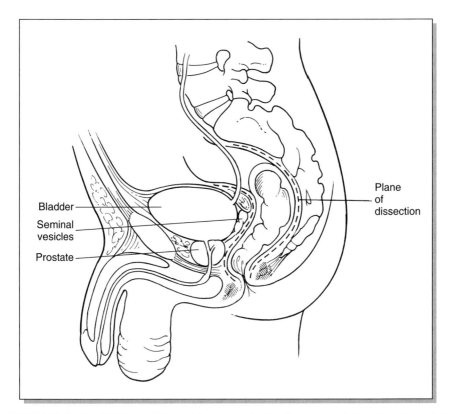

FIGURE 36–1   Sagittal view of the pelvis demonstrating the plane of dissection for rectal resection.

remove the mesorectum intact with its fascial envelope. This dissection is aided by retracting the rectum anteriorly with a malleable retractor. The loose areolar tissue between the mesorectum and presacral fascia is divided. After this, attention is directed to the anterior dissection. The peritoneal lining anteriorly is incised, and the bladder is retracted superiorly with a St. Mark's deep pelvic retractor to open the plane. Next, the Denonvilliers' fascia is incised, and the anterior rectal wall is separated from the seminal vesicles and the posterior capsule of the prostate. Laterally, the lateral stalks containing the middle hemorrhoidal vessels are clearly identified. While keeping the ureters under view, the lateral stalks are secured with large hemoclips and divided. Alternatively, the lateral stalks can be conveniently divided with the harmonic scalpel, particularly if access is difficult in a deep pelvis.

After completion of this circumferential dissection in the pelvis, the rectum should rise out of the pelvis and a distal margin of 5 cm is marked with a 2-0 silk suture, although 2 cm has been found to be adequate. Two traction sutures using 0-0 silk are placed on the lateral walls of the rectum. A right-angle occlusive clamp is placed proximal to this level, and the rectum is divided using a TA-55 reticulating stapler.

In preparation for the anastomosis, adequate mobilization, absence of tension, and blood supply of the descending colon are confirmed. A purse-string suture using 3-0 monofilament nonabsorbable suture is placed around the opening of the descending colon. The anvil of the EEA stapler is inserted into the descending colon and the purse-string suture is tied down. An end-to-end stapler, usually 28 to 30 Fr, is lubricated well and inserted through the predilated anal canal. The spike of the stapler is advanced just anterior to the distal staple line and engaged to the anvil that is placed within the proximal bowel (Fig. 36–2A). The stapler is closed and fired. After removal of the stapler, adequacy of the anastomosis is checked in several ways:

- The integrity of the two tissue doughnuts is confirmed by inspection.
- The anastomosis is inspected with a flexible sigmoidoscope (Fig. 36–2B).
- With the pelvis full with warm saline, air is instilled into the bowel with a sigmoidoscope; the presence of bubbles usually indicates a leak.

If absolute hemostasis has been achieved, there is no need for pelvic drain. For an ultra-low colorectal anastomosis or coloanal anastomosis, a temporary diverting loop ileostomy should be considered.

CLOSURE   Standard closure for the midline incision is used.

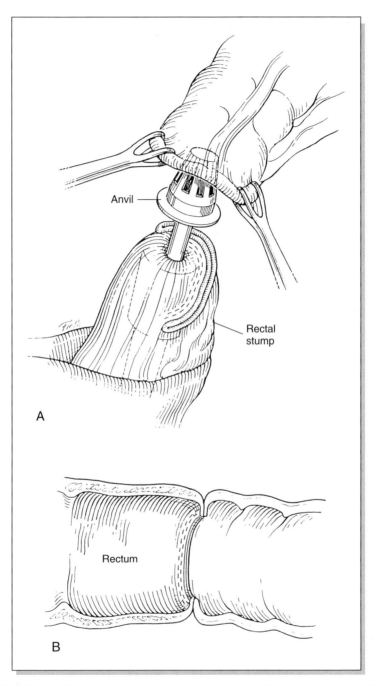

Anvil

Rectal stump

A

Rectum

B

FIGURE 36–2 *A,* After a low anterior resection the stapling device is used for the anastomosis. *B,* The completed anastomosis with a double staple line.

ABDOMINOPERINEAL RESECTION OF RECTUM

The preoperative preparation and the abdominal portion of the procedure are similar to those described for the anterior resection of the rectum; therefore, the perineal resection is described here.

Operative Procedure

PERINEAL DISSECTION   Start the perineal dissection by identifying the key anatomic landmarks: the perineal body, right and left ischial tuberosities, and coccyx. An elliptic incision extending from the perineal body to the coccyx is drawn with an indelible pen (Fig. 36–3A). The skin is incised with a no. 10 scalpel deepened down through the subcutaneous tissue. The perianal skin ellipse is grasped with three Allis clamps, and the subcutaneous tissue is further divided with electrocautery. Dissection proceeds directly down toward the coccyx. A moon-shaped incision is made at the tip of the coccyx, and the anococcygeal raphe is identified. The anococcygeal raphe is sharply divided with electrocautery. The Waldeyer fascia is encountered next and sharply divided to enter the presacral space. Laterally, the superficial fascia is divided to enter the ischiorectal fossa on both sides. The fat within the ischiorectal fascia is divided along the same furrow created on the lateral aspect. It is prudent to conceptualize the boundaries of the ischiorectal fossa:

- Laterally, the ischial tuberosity and the obturator fascia overlying the extrapelvic portion of the obturator internus
- Medially, the infra-anal fascia covering the levator ani and the sphincter ani muscles
- Ventrally, the transverse perinei superficialis and profundus muscles
- Dorsally, the fascia of the gluteus maximus muscle

In the upper part of the ischiorectal fossa, the inferior hemorrhoidal vessels are clamped, divided, and ligated with 2-0 absorbable sutures. Electrocoagulating these vessels must be avoided because they tend to retract, causing bleeding at a later point postoperatively. Once the ischiorectal fossa has been opened bilaterally, a self-retaining St. Mark's retractor is placed to facilitate further exposure. Posterior dissection is continued by elevating the anal canal with a malleable retractor and dividing the areolar tissue between the presacral fascia and the rectal fascia with electrocautery. The anal canal and then the rectum are progressively elevated from the presacral fascia, avoiding dissection too

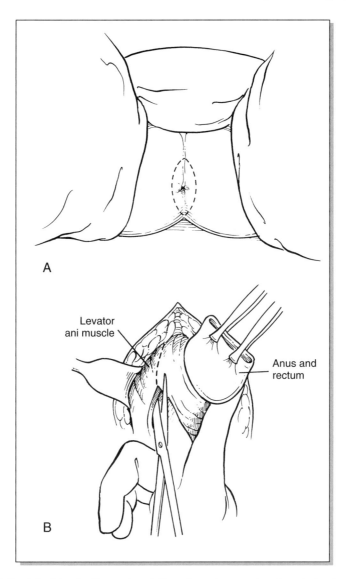

FIGURE 36–3 *A,* Incision for the perineal dissection when performing abdominoperineal dissection. *B,* The levator muscles are being divided with Metzenbaum scissors.

close to the sacrum because this can lead to troublesome bleeding from the presacral veins. Conversely, dissection too far anteriorly should be avoided to prevent risk of entering the rectum. If necessary, the abdominal operator should be allowed to direct the perineal dissector into the proper plane. In addition, it is important to keep a mental note of the curves of the rectum as the posterior dissection proceeds.

The index and middle fingers are passed beneath the iliococcygeus muscle on the right and then the left side, and the iliococcygeus muscles are divided sequentially with electrocautery or Metzenbaum scissors (Fig. 36–3*B*). The lateral dissection is continued ventrally by dividing the pubococcygeal muscle. The rectum still remains suspended by the puborectalis sling muscle. This muscle is placed under tension with the use of two malleable retractors in the lateral space, one laterally to retract the ischiorectal fat and the other medially over the rectum. The puborectalis muscles are divided in a longitudinal fashion on each side, thus allowing the rectum to fall dorsally. It is important to avoid drifting too far ventrally, because this may result in injury to the urethra. It is prudent to feel for the catheter within the urethra intermittently during this dissection. After the posterior dissection has been completed, the clamped sigmoid end of the operative specimen is drawn out through the posterior end of the perineal wound until the sigmoid and the upper two thirds of the rectum have been delivered out of the pelvic cavity.

The anterior dissection is now started. It is the most difficult portion of the perineal dissection because the rectum/anal sphincters are closely attached to membranous urethra, prostate, and seminal vesicles. The anterior skin is retracted while downward traction on the anal skin ellipse is applied to reveal the plane of dissection. The posterior border of the transverse perineal muscle is exposed. The rectourethralis is divided in the midline, and the plane between the rectum and the prostate is entered. The remaining anterior attachments are thinned by progressively dividing tissues on the sides. Again, it is important to palpate the Foley catheter and the prostate intermittently to avoid injury to these structures. Near the final stages of the dissection, it is important to support the rectum because it can be easily avulsed off the prostate or the urethra, which can result in inadvertent injury and troublesome bleeding.

The empty pelvic cavity is irrigated, and bleeding points are secured with a combination of electrocautery and suture ligatures using 2-0 absorbable sutures. If there is concern regarding hemostasis within the pelvis, it should be packed. Otherwise, two closed suction drains are placed in the pelvis and secured with 3-0 nonabsorbable sutures.

CLOSURE   The skin is approximated with interrupted mattress sutures using 3-0 monofilament nonabsorbable sutures.

CHAPTER 37

Construction and Reversal of Colostomy

A colostomy is an opening made into the large bowel to divert its contents to the exterior. The procedure is often part of another operation such as abdominal resection or subtotal colectomy or may be performed independently for bowel obstruction. It is uncommonly performed for colonic injuries.

PREOPERATIVE PREPARATION If colostomy is part of an elective bowel resection, preparation should be as for the primary procedure. The patient should be assessed preoperatively by the stoma therapist to be evaluated for the optimal placement of the stoma.

Operative Procedure

End Colostomy

EXPOSURE AND OPERATIVE TECHNIQUE The site of the stoma is selected; it should be approximately 10 cm from the anterior superior iliac spine and obliquely toward the umbilicus. Creases should be avoided, and in the presence of a panus, the stoma is placed higher up on the abdominal wall.

The linea alba is grasped with Kocher clamps, the site of the stoma is selected, and the skin is grasped with a

Kocher clamp. The Kocher is lifted and a circular skin incision is made. The dermis is incised with cutting electrocautery. A block of subcutaneous fat is excised, and using Army-Navy retractors dissection is continued until the anterior rectus sheath is visualized. The anterior rectus sheath is incised in a cruciate fashion. With Kelly or Rochester-Péan clamps, the rectus muscle is spread transversely and longitudinally to identify the posterior rectus sheath. A similar cruciate incision is made. The resulting defect in the anterior abdominal wall should easily admit two fingers. Two Babcock clamps are passed through the defect to grasp the colon and are gently drawn through the defect, avoiding any twists or constriction of the mesentery (Fig. 37–1A). The bowel is secured to the anterior rectus sheath at the four cardinal points with seromuscular bites using 3-0 silk sutures. If there is adequate length of mucosa, an attempt is made to rosebud the stoma; otherwise, it is secured flush to the skin using 3-0 absorbable sutures.

To rosebud the stoma, a bite of the dermis is taken, followed by a seromuscular bite of the adjacent bowel; the maneuver is completed by passing the suture through the full thickness of the edge of the bowel wall. Four such sutures are placed in the cardinal points and then tied down to evert the bowel. Using 3-0 absorbable sutures, additional sutures between the skin and the edge of the bowel are placed to completely secure the stoma (Fig. 37–1B).

To ensure that there is no obstruction secondary to any twisting of the colon, the stoma is gently examined with a lubricated finger. The skin around the stoma is cleansed and degreased with alcohol, and a stoma bag is placed.

Loop Colostomy

A loop colostomy may be constructed to divert fecal stream from an anastomosis. Alternatively, a loop colostomy can be created for a left colon obstruction on an emergent basis or permanently for palliating an unresectable cancer.

EXPOSURE AND OPERATIVE TECHNIQUE An 8- to 10-cm transverse incision is made approximately 2.5 cm above the umbilicus over the left half of the rectus sheath. The anterior rectus sheath and then the rectus muscle are divided with electrocautery. Larger blood vessels are clamped and ligated with 2-0 silk sutures because they often retract during electrocautery. The posterior rectus sheath is incised, and the peritoneal cavity is entered.

The transverse colon is identified by the teniae coli and delivered through the wound. In obese patients, to avoid retraction, the loop of

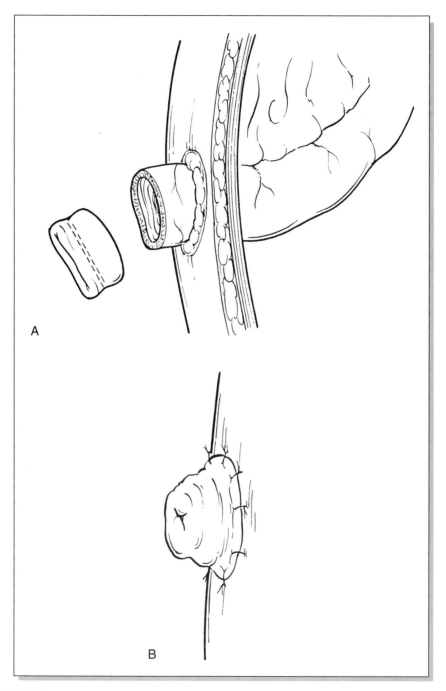

FIGURE 37–1 *A,* The loop of bowel is brought through a circular defect created in the anterior abdominal wall. *B,* The edges of the bowel wall are approximated to the skin.

transverse colon is suspended with rubber tubing or a glass rod. A small opening is made within the mesentery and the plastic T-piece is passed through this defect. The colon is secured to the anterior rectus sheath at four cardinal points with 3-0 silk sutures. The colon is opened transversely along the teniae and the contents suctioned. Using 3-0 absorbable sutures, the colostomy is secured by taking bites of all layers of the colonic wall and the dermis. If complete diversion is required, the transverse colon is divided with a GIA-60 stapler. The peritoneal covering of the mesentery is incised on both sides. The vessels in the mesentery are divided and ligated with 2-0 silk sutures. During this mobilizing maneuver, care should be taken to avoid compromising the blood supply of the colon. The proximal colon is then matured in the usual fashion. The distal mucous fistula is usually left closed unless there is fear of closed loop formation, in which case it is also matured.

CLOSURE   After constructing the colostomy, any remaining open abdominal incision is approximated in the usual fashion. Next, the colostomy bag is closed over the stoma.

Reversal of Loop Colostomy

PREOPERATIVE PREPARATION   It is recommended that at least a 3-month period elapse before contemplating closure of the colostomy. Furthermore, the patient should have recovered from the primary pathologic process that necessitated the construction of the temporary colostomy. The colon should be evaluated with either a barium enema or colonoscopy to ascertain the integrity and patency of the segments to be reconnected. The patient undergoes a standard mechanical bowel preparation. The remaining preparation is as described for other colonic procedures.

Operative Procedure

POSITION   The patient is placed in the supine position, and general anesthesia is provided.

INCISION   A circumferential incision at the mucocutaneous junction of the colostomy is made and can be extended on each side if further exposure is required (Fig. 37–2A).

EXPOSURE AND OPERATIVE TECHNIQUE   The incision is carried down through the subcutaneous tissue until the wall of the bowel is identified (Fig. 37–2B). If necessary, the colostomy edges can be closed together to prevent any

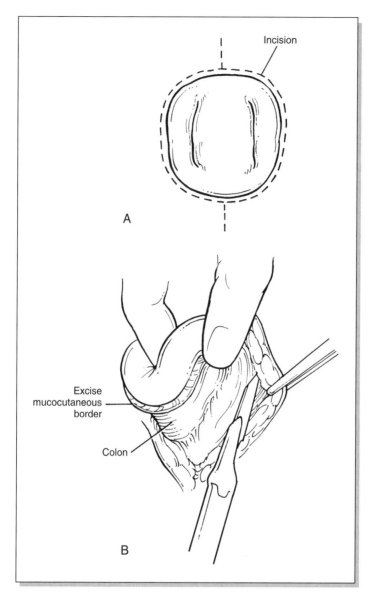

FIGURE 37–2 *A,* A circumferential incision is made at the mucocutaneous junction. *B,* The loop of bowel is dissected free from the subcutaneous tissue and the fascia.

Illustration continued on the following page

spillage. Alternatively, the colostomy can be left open and the surgeon can place a finger in the lumen to facilitate the identification of the bowel wall.

Dissection proceeds until the anterior abdominal fascia is identified. The loop of bowel is dissected free from the anterior abdominal wall, with particular care taken to identify the mesentery to avoid injury. The adhesions between the parietal peritoneum and the colon are divided by gentle dissection. After this mobilization, several centimeters of each limb should be exteriorized. If any difficulty is encountered, the fascial opening can be enlarged. Soft Doyen intestinal clamps are placed across the two limbs of bowel, with particular care taken to avoid any twisting of the colon limbs. The segment of colon containing the colostomy is resected.

A hand-sewn end-to-end anastomosis is constructed with two layers. First, the posterior layer of interrupted 3-0 silk Lembert sutures is placed. Next, an inner posterior row of 3-0 absorbable sutures is placed encompassing all layers of the bowel and converting to Connell sutures for the anterior inversion (Fig. 37–2C). At this point the Doyen clamps are

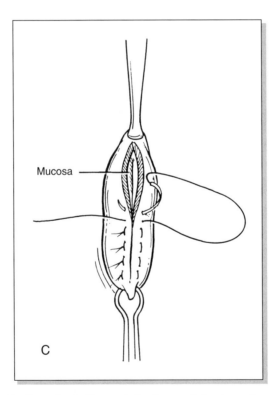

Mucosa

C

FIGURE 37–2 *Continued.* *C,* The anterior layer of the bowel anastomosis is being performed.

removed and the anastomosis is completed by placing the anterior row of interrupted seromuscular 3-0 silk Lembert sutures. The defect in the mesocolon can be closed with either continuous or interrupted 3-0 absorbable sutures, and the segment of bowel is returned to the abdominal cavity.

CLOSURE   The wound is irrigated with saline. The defect in the anterior abdominal wall is closed in layers. The peritoneum and the posterior fascia are closed together with continuous 0-0 monofilament nonabsorbable sutures, and the anterior fascia is approximated with 1-0 monofilament nonabsorbable sutures. The skin and subcutaneous tissue are left open and packed with saline-soaked gauze; delayed primary closure is performed on the fifth postoperative day. Alternatively, the skin can be approximated with a few staples.

CHAPTER 38

Hemorrhoidectomy

ANATOMY   Within the submucosa of the anal canal is a venous plexus that primarily drains into the superior rectal vein. It is through this venous plexus that the superior, middle, and inferior rectal veins communicate with each other. Internal hemorrhoids represent varicosities of the tributaries of the superior rectal vein that lie in the anal columns at the 3, 7, and 11 o'clock positions and are covered by mucous membrane. Therefore, a hemorrhoid is composed of a fold of mucous membrane and submucosa containing a varicosed tributary of the superior rectal vein and a terminal branch of the superior rectal artery. External hemorrhoids are varicosities of the tributaries of the inferior rectal vein that are covered by skin.

SPECIAL PREPARATION   Hemorrhoidectomy can easily be accomplished with sedation and local anesthesia or spinal anesthesia. The patient is administered an enema on the day of the surgery. Before performing a hemorrhoidectomy, the surgeon must be diligent to exclude important perianal pathology that requires alternative treatment modalities. These include anal and perianal squamous cell carcinoma; lymphoma in immunocompromised individuals; leukemic infiltration; and, finally, Crohn's disease, for which a conservative approach must be considered.

Operative Procedure

POSITION   The patient is placed in the jackknife position and the buttocks are separated with adhesive tape.

243

The perianal area is scrubbed and prepped with an antiseptic solution, and the patient is draped. The anal canal is gently dilated with two lubricated fingers, followed by placement of a self-retaining retractor. The anal canal is irrigated with Betadine solution while any remaining mucous or fecal material is suctioned.

EXPOSURE AND OPERATIVE TECHNIQUE The subcutaneous and submucosal planes are slowly infiltrated with a local anesthetic agent and massaged to spread this agent. Hemorrhoidal tissue present in the left midlateral, right posterolateral, and right anterolateral position is identified (Fig. 38–1A). Excision is begun with the right posterolateral hemorrhoid. The mucosa on each side of the hemorrhoid is incised and the incisions are extended outward toward the anoderm (see Fig. 38–1A). With fine curved scissors, the anoderm and the hemorrhoidal mass are elevated off the transverse fibers of the internal sphincter muscle (Fig. 38–1B). Dissection is continued just beyond the dentate line, the pedicle is clamped at the apex, and the hemorrhoidal tissue is excised. The pedicle of the hemorrhoid at

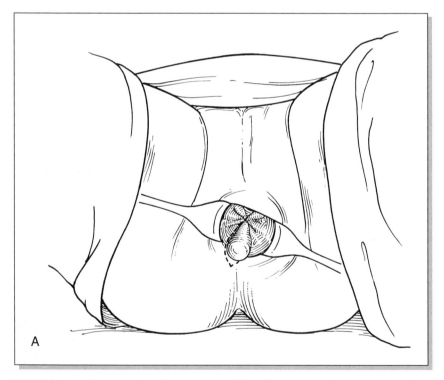

A

FIGURE 38–1 A, Hemorrhoidal tissues are identified. The mucosa is incised on each side of the hemorrhoid and extended outward toward the anoderm.

the apex is ligated with 2-0 absorbable sutures. Hemostasis is achieved. Then, starting at the apex, the mucosa is approximated with continuous 3-0 absorbable sutures (Fig. 38–1*C*). Intermittently, bites of the underlying internal sphincter are taken to allow the mucosa to adhere to it.

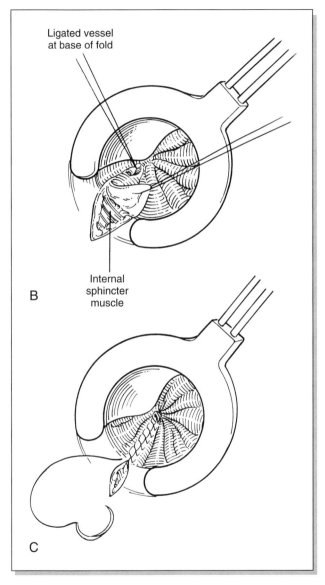

FIGURE 38–1 *Continued.* *B*, The anoderm and the hemorrhoidal mass are elevated off the transverse fibers of the internal sphincter muscle. *C*, The mucosa is approximated with continuous 3-0 absorbable sutures, leaving 2 to 3 mm of the anoderm left open for drainage.

Approximately 2 to 3 mm of the anoderm is left open for drainage. The same procedure can be performed for the other two hemorrhoidal masses.

Alternatively, the prolapsing hemorrhoids are identified and grasped. With fine curved scissors, the skin at the anal verge is incised and the hemorrhoidal tissue is elevated off the external sphincter. A clamp is placed at the base of the hemorrhoid, which is excised with a scalpel. A transfixing 3-0 absorbable suture is placed at the apex of the hemorrhoidal tissue and continued as an over-and-over continuous suture to approximate the mucosa. The remaining hemorrhoids are dissected in the same manner.

For large hemorrhoids, a single mucosal incision is made at the dome of the hemorrhoid, which is mobilized with submucosal dissection and excised. After this, the mucosa is reapproximated with 3-0 absorbable sutures. This method avoids resection of excessive mucosa, which could lead to anal stenosis. Likewise, excessive removal of anoderm should be avoided, because it is unnecessary and also can lead to anal stenosis.

At completion of the procedure, a bolster made of rolled gauze wrapped with lubricated petroleum jelly gauze is inserted into the anal canal. Finally, a dry gauze dressing is placed near the anal opening and can be removed postoperatively before the patient is discharged.

Vascular Surgery

CHAPTER 39

Repair of Abdominal Aortic Aneurysm

EMBRYOLOGY   Clusters of angiogenic cells form bilaterally on the lateral sides of the splanchnic mesoderm, close to the midline. These clusters acquire a lumen and form the paired longitudinal vessels, called dorsal aortae. Initially these are continuation of the endocardial heart tubes, but with rotation of the cardiogenic plate, the proximal portion of the dorsal aortae becomes arched. During development, the dorsal aortae fuse to form a single vessel just caudal to the branchial arches. Several intersegmental arterial branches carry blood to the somites and their derivatives. In the abdomen, most of the dorsal segmental arteries become the lumbar arteries, but the fifth pair of intersegmental arteries becomes the common iliac arteries. The caudal portion of the dorsal aorta becomes the median sacral artery.

ANATOMY   The aorta enters the abdominal cavity through the diaphragm at the level of the 12th thoracic vertebra. It lies anterior to the vertebral bodies and bifurcates into two common iliac arteries at the level of the fourth lumbar vertebra. Lying on its right side is the inferior vena cava. The cisterna chyli lies between the aorta and the inferior vena cava at the level of the diaphragm. On the left side lies the left sympathetic trunk. From above and downward, the aorta is covered anteriorly by the peritoneal lining of the lesser sac, the pancreas and the splenic vein, the left renal vein, the third part of the duodenum, and the loops of small bowel.

The branches of the abdominal aorta can be divided into the following groups:

- Anterior vessel branches: celiac axis, superior mesenteric artery, and inferior mesenteric artery
- Lateral vessel branches: suprarenal arteries, renal arteries, and gonadal arteries
- Parietal branches: the phrenic arteries and four paired lumbar arteries
- Three terminal branches: one median sacral artery and two common iliac arteries at the level of the sacroiliac joints dividing into the internal and external iliac arteries

PREOPERATIVE PREPARATION Once the decision has been made to electively repair an abdominal aortic aneurysm, pulmonary, renal, and cardiac function must be thoroughly evaluated. Pulmonary function tests are obtained, and preoperative therapy, including bronchodilators, is instituted if needed. Cessation of smoking is encouraged, and the patient is taught incentive spirometry. If there is clinical evidence of cardiac dysfunction, cardiac echocardiography and thallium stress tests are obtained to assess perfusion and ventricular function. Baseline, complete blood count, electrolytes, blood urea nitrogen, creatinine, and coagulation profiles are performed routinely. If a transabdominal aortic aneurysm repair is contemplated, the patient should be prepped with a modified Condon-Nichol bowel preparation.

Prophylactic antibiotics are administered. If preoperative cardiac work-up reveals ventricular dysfunction, the patient can be admitted preoperatively for insertion of Swan-Ganz catheter and optimization of cardiac function.

ANESTHESIA The patient undergoes general anesthesia. An epidural catheter can be placed for postoperative pain management. A urinary bladder catheter, a nasogastric tube, and radial arterial lines are placed.

Operative Procedure

POSITION The patient is placed in the supine position with both arms abducted at 90 degrees to allow access for the anesthesiologist. The lower chest, abdomen, and groin are scrubbed, prepped, and draped in sterile fashion.

INCISION A vertical midline incision extending from the xiphoid to pubis is made.

EXPOSURE AND OPERATIVE TECHNIQUE The abdominal cavity is entered in the usual fashion, and a thorough exploration is performed to exclude any unexpected lesions, particularly gastrointestinal malignancies. The patient is placed in a slight Trendelenburg position, and a self-retaining retractor system is arranged. The omentum and the transverse colon are retracted upward, and the small bowel is carefully packed in the right upper quadrant with the use of moist towels and appropriate retractors.

The peritoneal covering over the anterior surface of the aorta is opened using Metzenbaum scissors, and the opening is extended over both iliac arteries. Circumferential dissection is not required and is in fact not advised, because it may lead to injuries to the inferior vena cava and the iliac veins. Both ureters are identified and protected from injury. The extent of the aneurysm and the status of the iliac arteries are assessed, and a decision is made to proceed with either a simple tube graft or an aortic bifurcation graft.

The anesthesiologist is instructed to administer a 5000-unit bolus of intravenous heparin. After this, the iliac arteries are cross-clamped to prevent distal embolization. Attention is now directed to exposing the neck of the aneurysm proximally. Division of the ligament of Treitz and the inferior duodenal attachments greatly facilitates this procedure. This dissection is continued until the left renal vein is exposed. The renal vein can be retracted upward to expose the neck of the aneurysm. If necessary, the renal vein can be transected close to the inferior vena cava if the neck of the aneurysm extends beneath this vein. Dividing the renal vein close to the vena cava preserves drainage through the gonadal and adrenal veins. The inferior mesenteric artery is identified, is carefully dissected, and can be divided if necessary. If the inferior mesenteric artery is large and a major contributor to the blood supply of the left colon, it may need to be reimplanted.

After informing the anesthesiologist, the operator cross-clamps the aorta in an anteroposterior direction (Fig. 39–1*A*). A longitudinal arteriotomy is made along the aneurysm, and the aortic wall is opened like a book with horizontal incisions proximally and distally. The contents of the aneurysm, which includes atheromatous material and clots, are bluntly but meticulously extracted. Bleeding from paired lumbar arteries is controlled with figure-of-eight sutures using 2-0 polypropylene monofilament sutures (Fig. 39–1*B*). Because the posterior wall of the aneurysm is left undisturbed, bleeding from lumbar veins is minimized. Normally, if the distal aorta is not aneurysmal, a tube graft is an appropriate choice. If the aneurysm extends to the level of the bifurcation, the common iliac arteries are prepared in a similar fashion, leaving the posterior wall intact. Likewise, if the distal aorta and the iliac vessels are aneurysmal, a standard aortobifemoral graft should be chosen. In this case the orifices of both iliac arteries are closed from within using 2-0 polypropylene

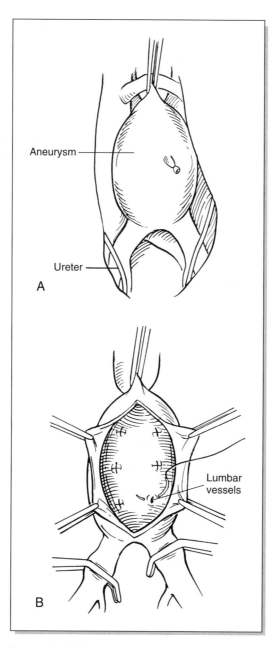

FIGURE 39–1 *A,* The neck of the aneurysm is cross-clamped below the renal vein. *B,* Bleeding from the lumbar arteries is controlled with figure-of-eight sutures.

monofilament sutures. The diameter of the nonaneurysmal area is measured, and an appropriately sized polytetrafluoroethylene (Gore-Tex) graft or a clotted knitted Dacron graft is chosen.

Proximal anastomosis is started with double-ended 2-0 polypropylene sutures that begin in the middle of the intact back wall of the aneurysm (Fig. 39–1*C*). Sutures are placed through the back wall of the aneurysm and then through the graft and continued until the lateral part of the graft is reached on both sides. From both sides the graft is sutured to the anterior wall of the aorta to meet in the midline anteriorly, where the sutures are tied down. The aorta is unclamped proximally, and any anastomotic leaks are controlled with figure-of-eight sutures using 3-0 polypropylene.

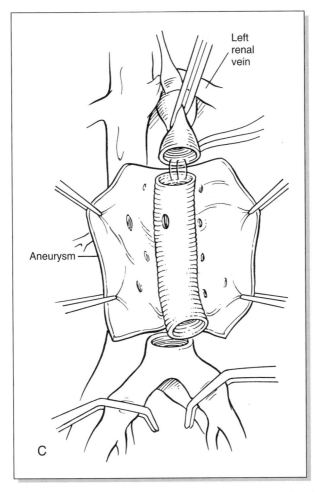

FIGURE 39–1 *Continued.* *C,* After the aneurysm is opened like a book, the graft is sutured. The renal vein can be seen retracted upward.

After the graft has been flushed, a long DeBakey clamp is placed across the graft. For the tube graft placement, the distal anastomosis to the aorta is performed in a similar manner. Alternatively, the limbs of the bifurcation graft are anastomosed to the common iliac arteries.

If an aortobifemoral graft is required, a separate team can expose the common femoral artery and its branches through an oblique incision in each groin. The two limbs of the Gore-Tex or Dacron graft are passed beneath the inguinal ligament in preparation for the distal anastomosis. An arteriotomy is made over the common femoral artery and extended toward the superficial femoral artery. An end-to-side anastomosis is constructed with 4-0 Gore-Tex or polypropylene monofilament sutures. Before completing the distal anastomosis, backbleeding is verified and the aortic graft is flushed. After the graft has been flushed to remove any clots, the clamps are carefully released and blood flow to the lower extremity is reestablished. The anesthesiologist must prepare for possible onset of hypotension before declamping. Once all the clamps have been released, topical hemostatic agents, such as Gelfoam and thrombin, can be placed around the anastomosis to promote hemostasis secondary to needle puncture leaks. Any brisk bleeding must be controlled with simple reinforcing sutures using 3-0 polypropylene.

CLOSURE The aneurysmal wall is reapproximated with 2-0 absorbable sutures. The peritoneum is reapproximated over the aorta, with care taken to avoid injury to the ureters. The small bowel is returned to the abdominal cavity. The area of the duodenum is carefully inspected, and the peritoneum is interposed between the graft and the duodenum to avoid development of aortoduodenal fistulas. The linea alba is closed with 1-0 polydioxanone. The skin is approximated with staples. If an aorto-bifemoral bypass has been performed, the groin incisions are closed in layers using 2-0 absorbable sutures. The skin is closed with staples.

CHAPTER 40

Femoropopliteal Bypass Grafting

EMBRYOLOGY   See Chapter 39.

ANATOMY   The common femoral artery is a continuation of the external iliac artery, and it enters the femoral triangle beneath the midpoint of the inguinal ligament. The femoral vessels are contained within the femoral sheath, which formed anteriorly from the transversalis fascia and posteriorly from the iliac fascia. This fascia blends with the adventitia of the femoral vessels approximately 3 cm below the inguinal ligaments. About 3 to 4 cm below the inguinal ligament, the profunda femoris artery arises from the lateral aspect of the common femoral artery. The common femoral artery continues obliquely downward as the superficial femoral artery. The superficial femoral artery exits the femoral triangle to enter the subsartorial canal and ends by passing through an opening in the adductor magnus to become the popliteal artery. From above downward, the femoral artery lies on the psoas tendon, which separates it from the hip joint and the pectineus and adductor longus muscles. In the femoral triangle the femoral vein lies medial to the femoral artery, and more distally in the subsartorial canal the vein lies posterior to the artery and maintains this relationship in the popliteal fossa. The femoral nerve and its branches are found lateral to the femoral artery.

Emerging from the fossa ovalis, several branches originate from the femoral artery: superficial circumflex iliac, superficial epigastric, and superficial external pudendal arteries. The deep external pudendal artery courses medially either behind or in front of the femoral vein to supply the scrotum/labium majus. The profunda femoris is a major branch that passes between the pectineus and the adductor longus to lie on the adductor brevis and magnus. After giving off the medial and femoral circumflex femoral arteries and three perforating branches, it ends as the fourth perforating artery. At the termination of the superficial femoral artery the paired descending genicular arteries originate, forming a rich collateral blood supply around the knee joint.

PREOPERATIVE PREPARATION   Patients undergo femoral popliteal bypass grafting for obliterative atherosclerosis of the femoropopliteal arterial segment, which leads to disabling intermittent claudication, distal gangrene, or ischemic ulceration. Patients with ischemic lower extremity symptoms are usually initially evaluated with noninvasive techniques such as duplex ultrasonography. However, before proceeding to arterial reconstruction, arteriography is essential to provide a "road map" for the operation, including the status of the collaterals, distal run-off, and reconstitution of vessels. A complete angiographic study should be obtained, including the infradiaphragmatic aorta extending down to both the tibial and peroneal systems. This allows appropriate evaluation of both inflow and outflow for the proposed graft. Magnetic resonance angiography should be obtained in patients who are unable to undergo arteriography secondary to renal impairment. Because these individuals generally have widespread vascular disease, the history and physical examination should also elicit any abnormality of cardiac, renal, and carotid systems if clinically indicated. Preoperative echocardiography and thallium stress/Persantine thallium tests should be obtained. Many of these patients are also heavy cigarette smokers; therefore, evaluating the respiratory system is crucial. The patients should be encouraged to stop smoking and advised on use of incentive spirometry. Diabetic patients should be encouraged to optimize their blood glucose levels. If the autologous saphenous vein is to be used as a conduit, this can be preoperatively marked in the vascular laboratory with the use of duplex ultrasonography. Preoperative antibiotics are administered.

Operative Procedure

ANESTHESIA   The procedure can be performed with either spinal or general anesthesia with endotracheal intubation.

POSITION   The patient is placed in the supine position, and the knee of the affected leg is flexed to 45 degrees with the hip also slightly flexed and externally rotated. Soft foam cushions or towels can be used to support the knee and the ankle. The lower abdomen and the affected leg are shaved, prepped, and draped in a sterile fashion. Operative time can be minimized if two surgeons work simultaneously.

Groin Exposure

INCISION   The femoral arteries are located approximately halfway between the pubic tubercle and anterior iliac spine. Just medial to this point, an oblique vertical incision is made (Fig. 40–1).

EXPOSURE AND OPERATIVE TECHNIQUE   The incision is carried through the skin, subcutaneous tissue, and superficial and deep fascia. A self-retaining Weitlaner retractor is placed. Dissection is carried directly toward the common femoral artery, which is dissected circumferentially, and a vessel loop is placed for control and to facilitate further mobilization of this vessel. Dissection proceeds proximally, the common femoral artery is identified and mobilized, and a vessel loop is placed around it. With the use of vessel loops, both the common and the superficial femoral arteries are elevated and displaced medially to bring the posterolaterally placed profunda femoris artery into view. The profunda femoris artery is also mobilized in a similar fashion and controlled by placing vessel loops (Fig. 40–2A).

Next, the greater saphenous vein is identified and dissected toward the saphenofemoral junction. All venous tributaries are ligated flush with the main femoral vein with 4-0 silk sutures. Once the saphenofemoral junction is exposed, a partially occluding curved vascular clamp such as a

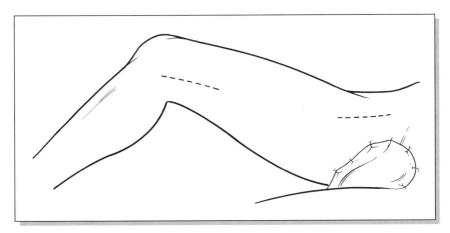

FIGURE 40–1   Incisions used for exposure of the femoral and popliteal vessels to perform femoropopliteal bypass.

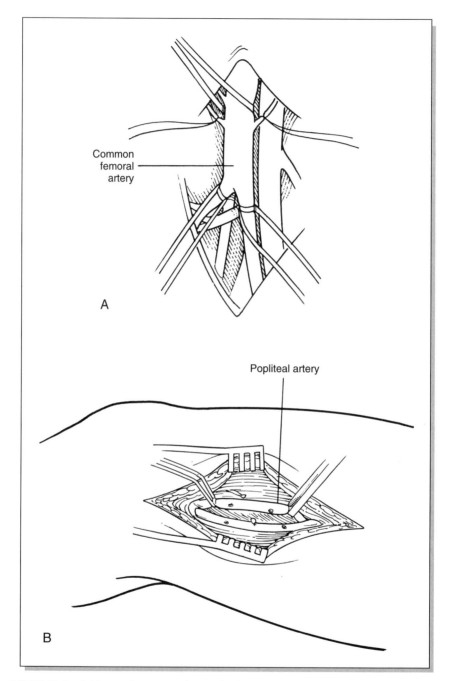

Common
femoral
artery

A

Popliteal artery

B

FIGURE 40–2   *A*, Exposed common femoral artery and its branches, superficial and profunda femoris artery. *B*, Exposure of the popliteal artery.

Satinsky is placed along the common femoral vein. The upper end of the greater saphenous vein is divided, along with a cuff of the common femoral vein. The common femoral vein is closed with continuous 3-0 polypropylene monofilament sutures, and the clamp is removed. The groin incision is extended distally directly above the course of the greater saphenous vein. If an in situ vein bypass is to be performed, attention is directed only at identifying the branches. These branches are ligated in continuity with 4-0 silk sutures.

Popliteal Exposure

INCISION   A 10- to 12-cm incision is placed just posterior to the border of the lower femur and along the long axis of the thigh (see Fig. 40–1). The popliteal artery is exposed above the knee if the artery appears to be of satisfactory quality at this site.

EXPOSURE AND OPERATIVE TECHNIQUE   For an above-knee approach, the incision is carried through the subcutaneous tissue and fascia. With the use of a self-retaining Weitlaner retractor, the sartorius is retracted superiorly. The upper popliteal artery is carefully freed from the adherent vein and dissected for a segment of approximately 5 cm. Vessel loops are placed at the two ends (Fig. 40–2*B*). The collateral vessels are controlled with 2-0 silk sutures.

If during the dissection this segment of the popliteal artery is noted to be thickened by atheroma, a below-knee approach is chosen. To expose the lower popliteal artery, an 8- to 10-cm incision is made approximately 1 cm behind the medial border of the tibia and parallel to the long axis of the lower leg. The subcutaneous tissues, superficial fascia, and deep fascia are incised in line with the skin incision. With the use of a self-retaining retractor, the medial head of the gastrocnemius is retracted posteriorly. The plane between the gastrocnemius and the popliteus is entered to expose the distal popliteal neurovascular bundle. To improve exposure, it may be necessary to divide the semimembranosus, the semitendinosus, the gracilis, and often the tendinous origin of the medial head of the gastrocnemius. Approximately 5 to 6 cm of the popliteal artery is exposed, and vessel loops are placed.

After the popliteal artery has been isolated, attention is directed toward dissecting the greater saphenous vein at this site. The tributaries of the greater saphenous vein are ligated with 4-0 silk sutures and divided. If an in situ vein bypass is contemplated, the tributaries of the greater saphenous vein are identified with the use of a Doppler probe. A small incision is made at this site. The tributaries are identified, carefully dissected, and ligated with 4-0 silk sutures. If a reverse saphenous vein bypass is to be performed, the entire length of the saphenous vein is harvested. The vein is gently distended with heparinized solution. Any additional branches are ligated with 4-0 silk sutures, and any small lacerations in the vein wall are closed with figure-of-eight sutures using 6-0 polypropylene monofilament sutures. Constricting adventitial bands are divided. To avoid twisting of the vein in the subfascial tunnel, the anterior surface of the vein is marked with a blue indelible pen. For in situ saphenous bypass, the venous valves need to be cut to allow downward flow. This can accomplished with a Leather valvulotome. The vein is gently flushed again with heparinized saline, and soft atraumatic bulldog clamps are placed at each end.

Essentially the same technique is used for all anastomoses. Before the proximal anastomosis is begun, the end of the greater saphenous vein is fashioned as an ellipse to create an oblique end-to-side anastomosis. The vessel loops around the common, superficial, and deep femoral arteries are tightened. With a no. 11 blade, a small arteriotomy is made on the anterior surface of the common femoral artery and extended using right-angle Pott scissors. Stay sutures using 4-0 polypropylene monofilament sutures are placed at the edges of the arteriotomy to improve exposure during the anastomosis. Two double-ended 4-0 polypropylene monofilament sutures are used to approximate the heel and the toe of the saphenous vein graft to the arteriotomy. The vein is sutured to the arterial wall in a continuous everting technique with the sutures placed approximately 2 mm apart. To avoid detaching the arterial intima, the needle is always passed first through the vein and then outward through the artery. The vessel loops are released, and the inflowing blood is allowed to flush through the distal end of the vein. A nontraumatic bulldog clamp is placed just distal to the completed anastomosis, and the vein is flushed with heparinized saline.

Next, preparation is made to perform the distal anastomosis in a similar end-to-side fashion using either 4-0 or 5-0 polypropylene monofilament sutures depending on whether an above-knee or a below-knee anastomosis is constructed. Just before the distal anastomosis is completed, backflow from the popliteal artery is checked. Then the bulldog clamp at the proximal anastomosis is released to establish inflow (Fig. 40–3). Any significant leaks are controlled with 5-0 polypropylene monofilament sutures. Flow in the popliteal artery is verified with palpation and with use of a Doppler probe. Intraoperative angiography should be performed at completion of the procedure.

If a prosthetic graft is being used as a conduit, it is tunneled, and the proximal and distal anastomoses are constructed in a similar fashion.

CLOSURE　　The wounds are irrigated, and the subcutaneous tissue of both incisions is closed with interrupted absorbable sutures. The skin is closed with staples.

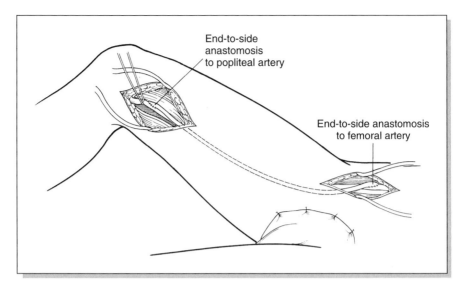

FIGURE 40–3 Completed femoropopliteal bypass showing the end-to-side proximal and distal anastomoses.

CHAPTER 41

High Ligation of Saphenofemoral Junction and Saphenectomy

ANATOMY The superficial veins of the lower extremity include the greater and lesser saphenous veins. The greater saphenous vein originates from the medial aspect of the dorsal venous arch and ascends anterior to the medial malleolus. It travels proximally on the medial aspect of the leg and the thigh within the subcutaneous tissues. In the groin region, the greater saphenous vein passes through the saphenous opening to join the femoral vein. Here it receives several venous tributaries such as the superficial circumflex iliac, superficial epigastric, and superficial external pudendal veins, which correspond to the branches of the common femoral artery at this location. The vein has numerous valves and also communicates with the deep venous system through a number of perforating veins present along the medial aspect of the thigh and calf.

The lesser saphenous vein originates from the lateral aspect of the dorsal venous arch and ascends posterior to the lateral malleolus along with the sural nerve. The vein travels along the middle of the calf, pierces the popliteal fascia, and passes between the two heads of gastrocnemius to end by entering the popliteal vein. The small saphenous vein too has numerous valves.

PREOPERATIVE PREPARATION   Patients with venous varicosities should have a careful physical examination and a review of the venous Doppler study to elicit the areas of incompetent perforators. If there is any evidence of cellulitis associated with ulceration, surgery should be postponed until the infection is resolved. Otherwise, standard evaluation of the cardiac, respiratory, and renal functions should be performed as indicated by the findings on history and physical.

Operative Procedure

POSITION   The patient is placed in the supine position. The procedure can be performed under either spinal or general anesthesia. The lower abdomen and the affected leg are prepped, and a stockinette is placed over the leg.

Ligation of the Saphenofemoral Junction, Ligation of Perforators, and Stripping of Varicose Branches

INCISION   The femoral pulse is palpated in the groin, and an oblique longitudinal incision is placed just medial to this point.

EXPOSURE AND OPERATIVE TECHNIQUE   The incision is carried down through the subcutaneous tissue with electrocautery, and the superficial fascia is incised. A self-retaining Weitlaner retractor is placed. The greater saphenous vein is identified and carefully dissected proximally toward the fossa ovalis. Here several venous tributaries will be seen entering into the great saphenous vein from both the medial and lateral aspects (Fig. 41–1A). These tributaries are ligated in continuity with 2-0 silk sutures and divided. The junction between the saphenous and the femoral veins is carefully dissected and exposed. Next, the greater saphenous vein is divided between clamps approximately 1 cm away from the saphenofemoral junction. The saphenofemoral junction is ligated with 0-0 silk sutures, and a 2-0 silk transfixion suture ligature is placed. Special care is taken not to narrow the femoral vein during this process. Careful inspection of the femoral vein is necessary to ensure that no other direct tributaries are left intact, because this can result in a recurrence of the lower extremity varicosities.

The next step depends on whether stripping of the greater saphenous vein is to be performed. Stripping of the greater saphenous vein can be avoided because the vein usually collapses and becomes sclerosed as long as the saphenofemoral junction and any incompetent perforators have been ligated. If stripping of the greater saphenous vein is to be performed, a Goldman vein stripper with the olive head at the distal end is gently passed through the open end of the great saphenous vein in the groin. If possible the stripper is passed down to the level of the ankle, where a transverse incision is made. The greater saphenous vein is isolated, divided, and ligated distally. The olive head is brought out through the vein at the ankle and secured with 0-0 silk sutures. Next, the stripper is pulled through the groin incision, thus stripping the varicosed greater saphenous vein. Alternatively, the Goldman vein stripper can be passed upward from the level of the ankle or the knee, such that the olive head emerges through the open end of the greater saphenous vein exposed in the groin (Fig. 41–1*B*).

The alternative method of addressing the varicosed venous branches is to ligate the preoperatively identified perforators in the thigh and the leg. The smaller varicosed tributaries that drain into the greater saphenous vein are avulsed. At the identified site of the perforators, a transverse

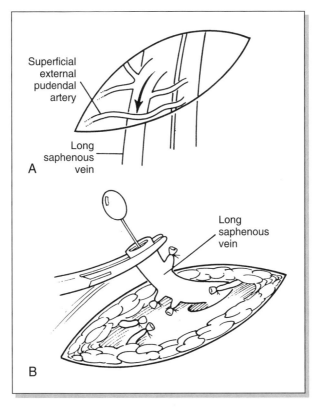

FIGURE 41–1 *A,* Saphenofemoral junction with tributaries entering the proximal aspect of the greater saphenous vein. *B,* The olive head of the Goldman stripper emerging through the open end of the greater saphenous vein in the groin.

skin incision is made. The varicosed greater saphenous vein is identified and elevated to visualize the communicating perforating vein. With a right-angle Mixter clamp, the perforated vein is carefully dissected and ligated with 2-0 silk sutures. The remaining perforators are addressed in the same fashion. Small tiny incisions are made over the small varicosed tributaries. These are lifted out of the wound using fine clamps and avulsed (Fig. 41–2). These small stab incisions can be closed with either Steri-Strips or a single interrupted 3-0 monofilament nonabsorbable suture.

CLOSURE   The groin incision is irrigated with saline and hemostasis secured. The superficial fascia is approximated with 3-0 absorbable sutures. The dermis is approximated with interrupted 3-0 absorbable sutures, and the skin is closed with subcuticular 4-0 absorbable sutures and is reinforced with Steri-Strips. The ankle incision from the stripping can also be closed with a few mattress sutures using 3-0 monofilament nonabsorbable sutures. The leg is wrapped with Kerlex gauze bandage and an elastic (Ace) wrap.

Ligation of the Saphenopopliteal Junction

INCISION   A transverse incision is placed along the popliteal fossa crease.

EXPOSURE AND OPERATIVE TECHNIQUE   On occasion, the lesser saphenous vein has evidence of varicosity and needs to be ligated. The patient is usually placed in the prone position to allow easy access to the popliteal fossa.

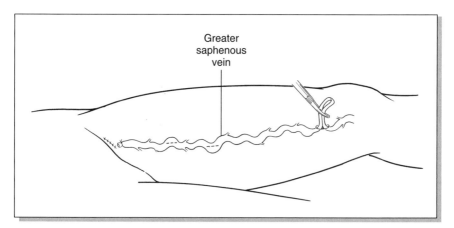

Greater
saphenous
vein

FIGURE 41–2 Through small stab incisions the varicosed veins are lifted out of the wound and avulsed.

A transverse skin incision is made and carried down through the subcutaneous tissue until the fascia is identified. The varicosed lesser saphenous vein is identified and followed through the fascia toward the popliteal vein. Small venous tributaries are ligated with 2-0 silk sutures and divided. The saphenopopliteal junction is carefully dissected while avoiding any injury to the adjacent popliteal artery and branches of the sciatic nerve. The short saphenous vein is divided between clamps and ligated with 2-0 silk sutures. A suture ligature of 3-0 silk is placed at the saphenopopliteal junction.

CLOSURE   The superficial fascia is approximated with 3-0 absorbable sutures. The dermis is approximated with interrupted 3-0 absorbable sutures, and the skin is closed with subcuticular 4-0 absorbable sutures and is reinforced with Steri-Strips.

CHAPTER 42

Lower Extremity Amputation

ANATOMY   Cross-sections of the lower extremity at the location of the incision greatly assist in recognizing the various muscles and neurovascular bundles encountered during the above- and below-knee amputations (Fig. 42–1).

PREOPERATIVE PREPARATION   Amputations are most commonly performed for peripheral vascular disease often associated with diabetes mellitus. Any extremity infection should be controlled and intravenous antibiotics administered. The patient's cardiac function should be assessed and optimized. In addition, the respiratory and renal systems should be evaluated. Patients who undergo amputation require a multidisciplinary approach and hence should be seen preoperatively by a physical medicine specialist, an occupational therapist, and an orthosis specialist. If the patient has diabetes, it too should be well controlled.

Operative Procedure

ANESTHESIA   Lower extremity amputations can be performed using spinal/epidural anesthetic or general anesthesia. Prophylactic antibiotics must be administered.

Above-Knee Amputation

POSITION   The patient is placed in the supine position, and the extremity and the lower abdomen are prepped

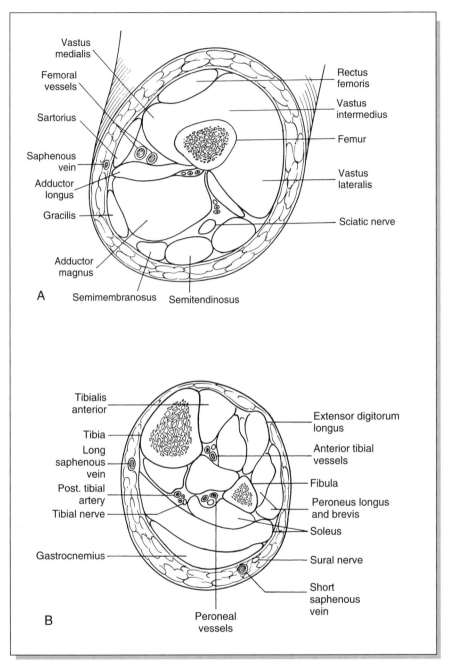

FIGURE 42-1 Cross-section of the lower extremity at the level of the thigh (A) and calf (B).

and draped such that the thigh and the knee are exposed. The knee is elevated with a kidney basin to gain access to the posterior structures of the leg.

INCISION Equal anterior and posterior skin flaps are outlined, with medial and lateral apexes 10 cm above the femoral condyles, such that the incision looks like a fish mouth (Fig. 42–2). The skin is incised sharply with a no. 10 scalpel, and the incision is carried through the subcutaneous tissue. The superficial veins encountered are divided and ligated with 2-0 silk sutures.

EXPOSURE AND OPERATIVE TECHNIQUE Medially, the superficial femoral artery and vein are located in the adductor canal, ligated, and divided with 0-0 silk sutures (Fig. 42–3A). The proximal stump of the vessels is further

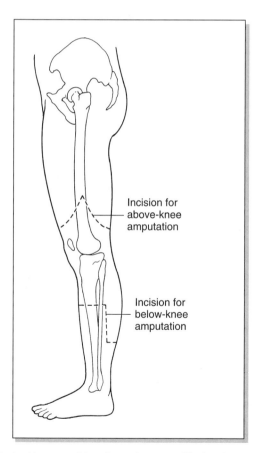

Incision for above-knee amputation

Incision for below-knee amputation

FIGURE 42–2 Incisions used for above-knee and below-knee amputations.

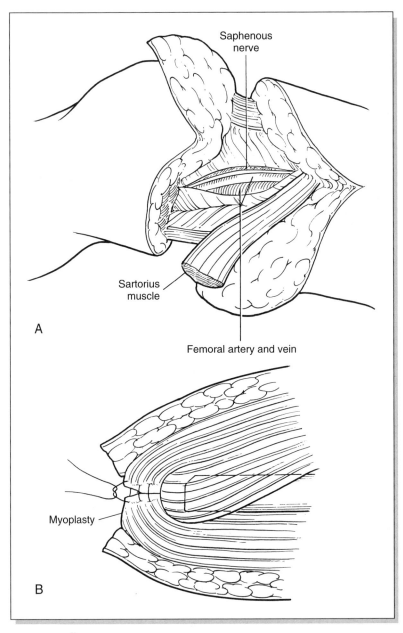

FIGURE 42–3 *A,* Identification of the femoral vessels and saphenous nerve after division of the sartorius muscle. *B,* Approximation of the divided muscles.

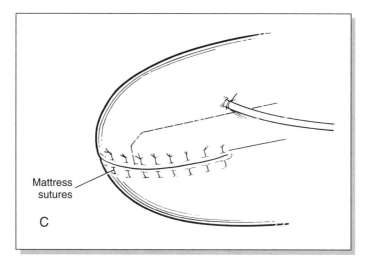

FIGURE 42–3 *Continued. C,* Skin closure with interrupted mattress suture after placement of a closed suction drain.

secured with transfixion suture ligatures using 2-0 silk sutures. The anterior flap is deepened through the quadriceps muscles toward the femur. Medially, the adductor magnus, adductor longus, and sartorius are divided with electrocautery. Laterally, the vastus lateralis, vastus intermedius, and tensor fasciae latae muscles are divided with electrocautery. The sciatic nerve should be ligated with 2-0 silk sutures, divided sharply, and allowed to retract. Next, the semimembranosus, semitendinosus, and biceps femoris muscles are divided with electrocautery. All bleeding muscular vessels are ligated with 2-0 absorbable sutures.

Next, the divided muscles are covered with moist laparotomy pads and retracted superiorly using Richardson retractors. The femur is divided approximately 10 cm above the femoral condyles with either a Gigli or a circular saw. The edges of the divided femur are smoothened with a bone rasper, and the filings are washed out with saline. Bleeding from the bone surface can be controlled with bone wax. Through separate stab incisions, suction drains are placed and directed within the deep muscle layers. The adductors are sutured loosely to the vastus lateralis and tensor fasciae latae over the femoral stump (Fig. 42–3*B*). Some surgeons use drill holes in the bone end to anchor the muscles to stop them from slipping off the femur. The deep fascia of the anterior and posterior flaps is approximated with 2-0 absorbable sutures.

CLOSURE   Once the myoplasty has been completed, the subcutaneous tissue is closely approximated with interrupted 2-0 absorbable sutures.

The skin is closed with interrupted mattress sutures using 3-0 nonabsorbable sutures, with particular care taken to handle the skin gently (Fig. 42–3C). The stump is bandaged with heavy dressing to protect the wound.

Below-Knee Amputation

POSITION   The entire leg is prepped and draped. The foot and lower part of the leg are covered with a stockinette. If the blood supply to the flaps is poor, the surgeon must be prepared to convert the procedure to an above-knee amputation.

INCISION   The anterior skin flap is outlined 10 cm below the tibial condyle and measures two thirds of the diameter of the leg (see Fig. 42–2). The longer posterior flap starts 20 cm below the tibial condyle and measures one third of the diameter of the leg. The skin is incised with a no. 10 scalpel, and the incision is extended through the subcutaneous tissue. Superficial veins are ligated with 2-0 silk sutures as they are encountered.

Viability of the flaps must be assessed by observing bleeding from the skin edges; if this seems to be inadequate, the procedure is converted to an above-knee amputation.

The incision is continued through the anterior compartment and its muscles, which include tibialis anterior, extensor hallucis longus, and extensor digitorum longus, which are sharply divided with electrocautery. The anterior tibial vessels are isolated with a right-angle Mixter clamp, doubly ligated with 2-0 silk sutures, and divided. These vessels are also transfixed with 3-0 silk suture ligatures.

EXPOSURE AND OPERATIVE TECHNIQUE   The tibia is divided transversely at the level of the anterior flap using a Gigli or a circular saw. An anterior bevel is cut and should be filed until absolutely smooth and rounded (Fig. 42–4A). The fibula is divided 1 to 2 cm above the level of the division of the tibia. The operative site is thoroughly lavaged. Laterally, the peroneal muscles are divided at the same level as the fibula. The peroneal vessels encountered are ligated and divided.

The posterior tibial vessels are identified, individually ligated, and divided (Fig. 42–4B). The plane between the tibialis posterior and the gastrocnemius–soleus muscle complex is entered; the latter muscles remain with the posterior flap. The tibialis posterior, flexor digitorum longus, and flexor hallucis longus muscles are individually divided with electrocautery. The deep veins of the calf are ligated with 2-0 silk sutures as they are encountered. To avoid a bulky stump, the muscles of the

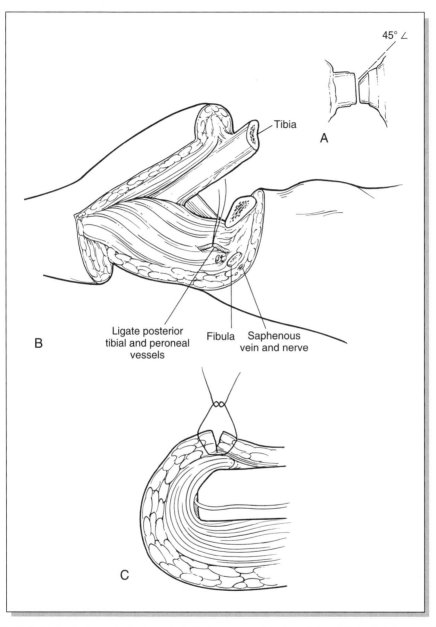

FIGURE 42–4 *A,* An anterior bevel of 45 degrees cut in the divided tibia. *B,* Division of the posterior tibial vessels after the tibia and fibula have been divided. *C,* Skin closure of the stump.

posterior flap are trimmed. The wound is irrigated with warm saline. The posterior skin flap is trimmed to match the anterior flap. Jackson-Pratt drains are placed within the muscle bed through separate stab incisions.

CLOSURE The deep fascia of the posterior flap is sutured to the deep fascia and periosteum of the anterior flap with 2-0 absorbable sutures. The skin is carefully approximated with interrupted mattress sutures using 3-0 nonabsorbable sutures (Fig. 42–4C). The stump is bandaged, as described for the above-knee amputation.

CHAPTER 43

Carotid Endarterectomy

EMBRYOLOGY   As the branchial arches develop during the fourth week, the aortic sac gives rise to six paired branches known as aortic arches. These aortic arches curve around the pharyngeal gut to terminate in the dorsal aortae of the corresponding side. The aortic arches are not present all at the same time, but they undergo complex modification and regression to result in the adult arterial arrangement by the eighth week of gestation. The proximal portion of the third aortic arch gives rise to the common carotid arteries, and their distal portion joins with the dorsal aortae to form the internal carotid artery. The external carotid artery is thought to be a branch of the third aortic arch.

ANATOMY   The right common carotid artery arises from the innominate artery, and at the level of the upper border of the thyroid cartilage it divides into external and internal carotid arteries. On the left side, the artery arises from the aortic arch and bifurcates into its terminal branches at the same level. At the proximal portion of the artery before its bifurcation, there is a dilatation called the carotid sinus (carotid bulb). The adventitia of the carotid sinus contains nerve endings from the glossopharyngeal nerve that are responsible for blood pressure regulation. The carotid body is a small neurovascular structure lying posterior to the carotid sinus that functions as a chemoreceptor. Each artery lies within the carotid sheath along with the internal jugular vein placed laterally and the vagus nerve posteriorly. Anterolaterally, the carotid sheath is covered by the sternocleidomastoid and the strap muscles. The trachea and the esophagus are present on the medial aspect of the carotid sheath.

The internal carotid artery ascends toward the base of the skull and enters the middle cranial fossa through the carotid canal at the foramen lacerum in the petrous temporal bone. It has no branches in the neck. The external carotid artery travels upward in the neck, first anteromedial and then lateral to the internal carotid artery. The styloglossus and stylopharyngeus muscles and the glossopharyngeal nerve separate these two terminal branches. The external carotid artery is crossed, from above downward, by the stylohyoid muscle, posterior belly of digastric muscle, hypoglossal nerve, and facial vein. The branches of the external carotid artery, in order of origin, include superior thyroid, ascending pharyngeal, lingual, facial, occipital, posterior auricular, superficial temporal, and maxillary arteries.

PREOPERATIVE PREPARATION   Patients with atherosclerotic carotid disease frequently have associated coronary artery disease; therefore, noninvasive evaluation of the cardiovascular system is essential. If necessary, coronary artery bypass grafting and carotid endarterectomy may be performed simultaneously. Preoperative pulmonary toilette teaching is advisable for patients who are smokers. The carotid color duplex study and angiogram are obtained to evaluate the extent of atherosclerotic disease. Prophylactic antibiotics should be administered. The patient generally undergoes general anesthesia, although some surgeons prefer to perform the procedure with the patient under local anesthesia to assess the patient's verbal communication and thus provide a continuous assessment of neurologic status. An arterial line is placed for continuous blood pressure monitoring. Agents to control hypertensive and hypotensive states should be readily available.

Operative Procedure

POSITION   The patient is placed in the supine position with the head resting on a foam doughnut ring. A folded sheet is placed beneath the shoulders to extend the neck. The head is turned away from the side that is being operated. The neck and the upper part of the thorax are prepped and draped in a sterile fashion.

INCISION   An oblique longitudinal incision is made along the anterior border of sternocleidomastoid muscle extending from the mastoid process to the medial aspect of the clavicle (Fig. 43–1).

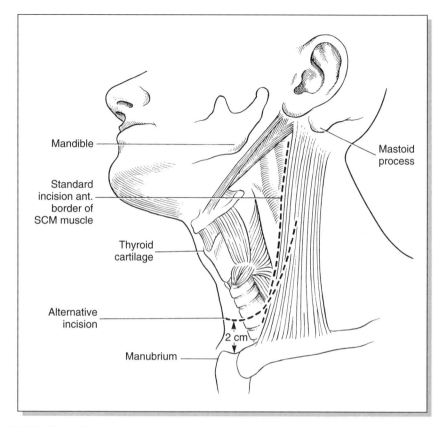

FIGURE 43–1 Standard incision along the anterior border of the sternocleidomastoid (SCM) muscle.

EXPOSURE AND OPERATIVE TECHNIQUE The skin, subcutaneous tissues, and platysma muscle are divided with electrocautery. At the superior part of the incision, the greater auricular nerve is identified and preserved. The deep cervical fascia is divided along the line of the incision, and a self-retaining Weitlaner retractor is placed to hold the sternocleidomastoid muscle posteriorly. The common facial vein is identified, clamped, divided, and ligated with 3-0 silk sutures to expose the carotid sheath. The carotid sheath is meticulously opened longitudinally, and the internal jugular vein is dissected laterally to allow access to the carotid artery. The common carotid and both the internal and external carotid arteries are carefully exposed using a meticulous combination of sharp and blunt dissection (Fig. 43–2). The hypoglossal and vagus nerves are identified and preserved. The ansa hypoglossi is usually transected to facilitate exposure and allows the hypoglossal nerve to be gently retracted out of the operative field.

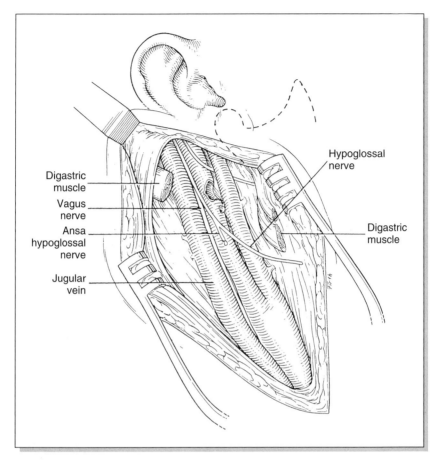

FIGURE 43–2 The common carotid and both the internal and external carotid arteries are carefully exposed. The hypoglossal nerve with the divided ansa hypoglossi and the vagus nerve can be seen.

The carotid sinus area is infiltrated with 1% lidocaine to prevent hypotension and bradycardia. Vessel loops are carefully passed around the common, internal, and external carotid arteries. The distal internal carotid artery is freed for at least 1 cm beyond the plaque. It is important to manipulate these vessels gently during the dissection to avoid embolization of atheroma. Systemic heparin embolization is established with an intravenous bolus of 5000 units of heparin. After 3 minutes, vessel loops around the common, internal, and external carotid arteries are tightened. Alternatively, vascular clamps may be used.

An arteriotomy is made with a no. 11 blade on the anterior wall of the common carotid artery and is extended into the internal carotid artery using right-angle Pott scissors. The use of a shunt is controversial. Some surgeons prefer to use the shunt routinely; others are selective and measure the internal carotid stump pressure to determine whether a shunt is necessary. A shunt is believed to be necessary if the internal carotid pressure is less than one third that of the radial artery pressure. A preprepared, appropriately sized shunt (Pruitt-Inahara or Javid shunt) is first inserted into the internal carotid artery, and the blood is allowed through backflow to fill the shunt. The proximal end of the shunt is then placed into the common carotid artery. The vessel loop around the internal artery is removed and replaced by a Javid clamp.

With the intraluminal shunt in place and cerebral blood restored, endarterectomy can commence. An appropriate plane, usually within the media, is carefully selected and developed in the common carotid artery with a Freer spatula. To facilitate the endarterectomy, the proximal plaque is transected with fine scissors, and the endarterectomy is continued distally. The plaque is first dissected out of the external carotid artery. In the internal carotid artery the plaque usually feathers out quite smoothly such that intimal flaps should not be created. If intimal flaps are present, they are carefully tacked down with U-shaped 6-0 polypropylene monofilament sutures. The inner lining of the exposed arteriotomy is gently flushed with heparinized saline. The arteriotomy is closed with continuous 6-0 polypropylene monofilament sutures; alternatively, if the vessel is believed to be narrow, a patch of polytetrafluoroethylene (Gore-Tex) or preferably a vein can be used.

Just before closing, the shunt is removed. The clamps are removed sequentially, allowing for flushing of these vessels—first the external, then the common, and finally the internal carotid arteries. This order minimizes the likelihood of cerebral embolization by allowing any loose fragments to instead travel into the external carotid artery. Blood flow is confirmed with a Doppler probe. Hemostasis from the suture line at the arteriotomy site can be achieved with placement of hemostatic agents such as Gelfoam and thrombin. Any areas of vigorous bleeding to the arteriotomy are controlled with figure-of-eight sutures using 6-0 polypropylene. Protamine sulfate can be administered to reverse heparinization if needed.

CLOSURE Through a separate stab incision, a 7-mm Jackson-Pratt drain is placed and secured with 3-0 nylon monofilament sutures. The platysma and then the subcutaneous tissue are carefully approximated with continuous 3-0 absorbable sutures. The skin is approximated with staples or closed with a subcuticular running 4-0 absorbable suture.

CHAPTER 44

Femoral Embolectomy

PREOPERATIVE PREPARATIONS Once the clinical diagnosis of lower extremity ischemia secondary to an embolus has been made, the patient is fully heparinized with 10,000 units intravenously as a bolus followed by a continuous infusion. Judicious fluid resuscitation and correction of electrolytes are necessary. A careful history and appropriate investigations are initiated to exclude cardiac dysrhythmias or acute myocardial infarction. Supplemental oxygen is provided with either a nasal cannula or a facemask.

ANESTHESIA If there are no contraindications owing to comorbid conditions, the procedure may be performed under general anesthesia with endotracheal intubation. Alternatively, arterial exploration may be undertaken under local anesthesia and accompanying sedation. Prophylactic antibiotics are administered. The abdomen, both inguinal areas, and the affected lower extremity are prepped and draped in a sterile fashion.

Operative Procedure

INCISION A longitudinal incision is made over the site of the common femoral artery, which is usually found midway between the symphysis pubis and the anterior superior iliac spine.

EXPOSURE AND OPERATIVE TECHNIQUE   The skin incision is carried through the subcutaneous tissue. A self-retaining Weitlaner retractor is placed. Because lymphatics are abundant in this area, lymph vessels should be ligated or controlled with small hemoclips. Using sharp dissection the common, superficial, and profunda femoris arteries are exposed. Vessel loops are placed around these arteries. The embolus frequently lodges at the bifurcation of the common femoral artery, and therefore a pulse may be palpable proximally but not distally. If a pulse is present, it may not be strong. It is important to recognize that a soft or a fully organized clot can transmit pulsation.

By applying traction on the vessel loops or by placing vascular clamps, the common femoral artery and its branches are occluded. Using a no. 11 scalpel, a small longitudinal arteriotomy is made on the anterior surface of the common femoral artery just above the origin of the profunda and is extended down to the superficial femoral artery with Pott scissors (Fig. 44–1A). The arteriotomy should be long enough to allow removal of

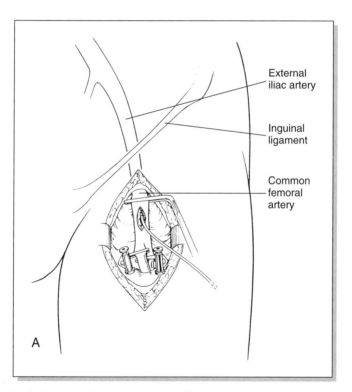

External
iliac artery

Inguinal
ligament

Common
femoral
artery

A

FIGURE 44–1   *A,* Common femoral artery and the terminal branches are controlled with vascular clamps. A Fogarty embolectomy catheter is passed proximally through the arteriotomy.

the embolus with ease. To keep the arteriotomy widely open during the embolectomy, gentle traction sutures may be placed at the edge of the arterial wall using 4-0 or 5-0 polypropylene and secured with a rubber-shod hemostat. Fogarty embolectomy catheters of various sizes must be available to extract the embolus from the proximal and distal aspect of the lower extremity arteries (Fig. 44–2A).

A Fogarty embolectomy catheter is passed proximally for about 30 cm to ensure that it has entered the aorta. The balloon is inflated and the catheter gently withdrawn. Because the balloon engages in the common iliac artery, it is often necessary to slightly deflate the balloon to avoid intimal damage (Fig. 44–2B). The surgeon, rather than the assistant, should control the balloon pressure during withdrawal of the embolectomy catheter. The embolus is removed, and a second pass with the Fogarty catheter in the proximal direction is made to remove any residual embolus. A vigorous blood flow should follow clearance of the clot, and then heparinized saline is injected into the common femoral artery and the vessel loop tightened to achieve proximal vascular control.

The Fogarty embolectomy catheter is now passed distally in the superficial femoral artery as far as it can travel and then withdrawn with the balloon inflated. Fragments of embolus and clot appearing at the arteriotomy are gently removed, and a second pass down the common femoral artery is made to remove any residual clot. The presence of vigorous retrograde blood flow indicates distal patency. Heparinized saline is flushed into the superficial femoral artery, and the vessel loop is tightened to secure distal vascular control. A similar maneuver is now performed in the profunda femoris artery and its patency confirmed with the backflow.

The arteriotomy is closed with 4-0 continuous polypropylene sutures. Before completion of the suture line, a small quantity of blood is flushed from each of the vessels by intermittently releasing the vessel loops. This has the additional benefit of displacing any clot that might have formed after the embolectomy. If the artery is small, a vein patch may be needed to avoid narrowing of the vessel lumen. Once all the vessel loops have been released, distal pulses are checked. Hemostasis is achieved.

CLOSURE The subcutaneous tissue is approximated in layers using 3-0 absorbable sutures, and the skin is approximated with staples. If the duration of ischemia exceeds 6 hours, it is wise to also perform a four-compartment fasciotomy. The purpose of the fasciotomy is to lower the pressure within the fascial compartments of the leg. This involves making two longitudinal incisions, one on the medial and the other on the lateral aspect, dividing the deep fascia covering all four compartments. This allows the edematous muscle to bulge into the subcutaneous compartment. The muscle viability must be checked. The wounds are dressed with moist sterile gauze and lightly wrapped.

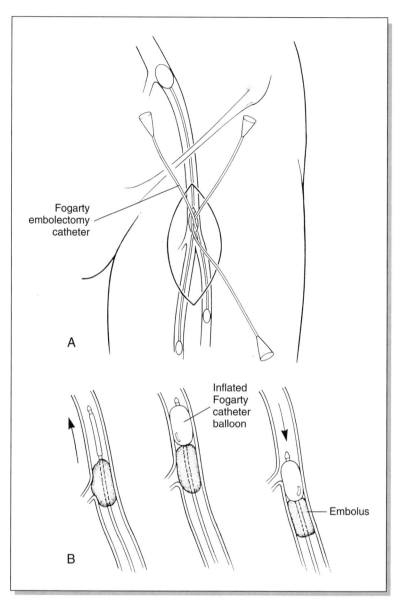

FIGURE 44–2 *A,* Fogarty embolectomy catheters of various sizes should be available to perform embolectomy. *B,* The balloon is inflated and the catheter is withdrawn to dislodge and remove the embolus.

Urology

CHAPTER 45

Nephrectomy

EMBRYOLOGY The genitourinary system is derived from the intermediate mesoderm and shows three stages of development:

1. *Pronephros:* Develops during the third week but is a nonfunctional system, and by the fourth week all the indications of the pronephric system have disappeared.

2. *Mesonephros:* Develops during the fourth week and replaces the vestigial pronephros. It functions as an interim structurally simple kidney until the permanent kidneys are formed from the metanephros (see below).

3. *Metanephros:* Develops during the fifth week of gestation and forms the permanent kidney, which arises in the lower lumbar and sacral regions.

At the terminal end of the mesonephric duct, an outgrowth called the ureteric bud appears and ascends along the pathway by which the mesonephric duct had descended. The ureteric bud penetrates the metanephros (condensation of mesoderm), which forms the metanephric cap. The distal end of the ureteric bud subsequently dilates, forming the primitive pelvis. Simultaneously, the primitive pelvis splits into cranial and caudal portions that divide and further subdivide to give rise to major and minor calyces. At the blind end of the minor calyces, collecting ducts are formed. At the distal end of the collecting ducts there is a metanephric tissue cap that under the influence of the tubule moves laterally to form renal vesicles. At the medial end, the vesicle becomes associated with the collecting tubule and breaks into it. The lateral end is invaginated by a small capillary loop, thus forming Bowman's capsule. The rest of the vesicle forms the proximal and distal convoluted tubules and the loop of Henle, thus resulting in a functioning kidney. The metanephros, which is initially located in the kidney, later ascends to a more cranial position—the ascent of the kidney. This migration is thought to occur due to diminution of the body curvature and the increased growth in the lumbar and the sacral regions. The metanephros derives its blood supply from the common iliac artery and subsequently directly from the aorta as the kidney ascends. The lower vessels degenerate, although they may persist as supernumerary renal arteries. Initially, the renal hilum is directed ventrally, but as the kidney ascends it rotates medially and the hilum points anteromedially.

ANATOMY   Both kidneys are retroperitoneal organs that lie on the posterior abdominal wall. The kidney and the associated structures are outlined in Figure 45–1. Each kidney lies obliquely, with the upper pole being nearer to the midline than the lower pole. Because of the presence of the liver on the right side, the right kidney is located slightly lower than the

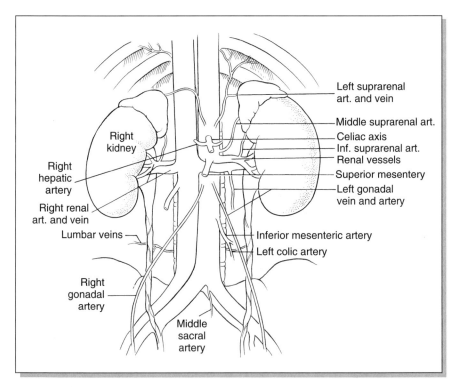

FIGURE 45–1   Anatomy of the kidney and the associated structures.

left. On the medial aspect of each kidney is the hilum, which is located approximately at the level of the transpyloric plane. Present at the hilum are the following structures, starting from the most superficial: the renal vein, the renal artery, and the ureter. The kidney has its own fibrous capsule but lies surrounded by perinephric fat that has an outer layer of perinephric fascia, known as Gerota's fascia. Gerota's fascia is a continuation of the transversalis fascia and separates the kidney from the adrenal glands that are located on the superior pole. The renal bed is composed of the diaphragm, the costal diaphragmatic recess of pleura, and the 11th and 12th ribs. The inferior aspect of the renal bed is formed by the psoas, quadratus lumborum, and transversus abdominis muscles. The three nerves that lie posteriorly to the kidney are the subcostal, iliohypogastric, and ilioinguinal nerves. Each renal artery arising from the aorta divides into several branches and supplies the kidney. The renal veins drain into the inferior vena cava, the right renal vein being much shorter than the left. The other veins that drain directly into the left renal vein include the left gonadal, left adrenal, and renolumbar veins. The lymphatic drainage is into the para-aortic nodes along the origin of renal arteries.

PREOPERATIVE PREPARATION A thorough assessment of the patient's cardiovascular and respiratory condition is performed. To evaluate contralateral renal function, baseline serum creatinine and, if necessary, a nuclear renal scan are obtained. Renal tumors are now commonly detected as an incidental finding on computed tomography of the abdomen. If nephrectomy is being performed for renal malignancy, the computed tomography scan or magnetic resonance image is carefully examined for the presence of renal vein or inferior vena cava tumor thrombus that would require special intraoperative approaches. If the patient is noted to have an elevated serum creatinine after contrast studies, intravenous fluid administration is indicated along with mannitol. If there is possibility of en bloc bowel resection, standard bowel preparation is necessary.

Operative Procedure

The approach to the kidney depends on the indication for nephrectomy. A simple nephrectomy for benign processes can be approached through the flank, whereas a radical nephrectomy for renal malignancy should be performed via a transabdominal approach.

Simple Nephrectomy

POSITION The patient is placed in a lateral position with the flexion of the operating table in line with the anterior superior iliac spine of the pelvis.

The lower leg is flexed to 90 degrees at the knee to prevent the body from rolling from side to side, whereas the upper leg is kept straight to maintain tension in the flank region. An axillary roll is placed under the lower dependent arm to prevent pressure on the axillary neurovascular bundle. The upper arm is placed on a special rest and secured. The lateral position of the patient is maintained by applying wide adhesive tape extending from the operating table and across the iliac crest. Another tape is placed at the level of the shoulder in a similar fashion to prevent the upper body from tilting forward. Next, the kidney rest is elevated and the operating table flexed, thus allowing the flank region to be under tension. All regions of the patient's body are carefully inspected, with particular attention to areas of pressure that must be relieved by placement of pillows. A nasogastric tube and Foley catheter are placed. The operative area is prepped and draped in the usual sterile fashion.

INCISION   The 12th rib is identified, because this will be the line of incision, starting over the rib and extending anteriorly up to the lateral border of rectus abdominis muscle.

EXPOSURE AND OPERATIVE TECHNIQUE   The incision is carried down sharply through the skin and subcutaneous fat until the 12th rib is visible along the posterior aspect of the incision. The external and internal oblique muscles are incised with electrocautery (Fig. 45–2A) to expose the dense lumbar dorsal fascia, which lies anteromedial to the tips of the 11th and 12th ribs. More medial to the lumbar fascia lies the transversus abdominis muscle. The lumbar dorsal fascia is opened, and two fingers are inserted beneath the transversus abdominis muscle to develop the extraperitoneal plane of dissection. As the peritoneum is reflected medially, the transversus abdominis muscle can be divided, and this dissection is continued toward the lateral margin of the rectus fascia. Posterior exposure is achieved by dividing the latissimus dorsi and serratus posterior muscles (see Fig. 45–2A). The diaphragmatic and intercostal muscle attachments to the 12th rib remain to be released. This can be achieved either by resecting the 12th rib or by carefully dividing the diaphragmatic attachments and the external and internal intercostal muscles. The wound is protected with laparotomy pads, and a self-retaining retractor is placed.

Using both digital and blunt dissection with a sponge stick, Gerota's fascia is separated medially off the psoas muscle. Gerota's fascia is incised and extended longitudinally. With a combination of blunt and sharp dissection, the perirenal fat is freed from the surface of the kidney. The kidney is mobilized forward to provide access to the posterior aspect of the hilum where the renal vessels are secured. The renal artery is identified and carefully dissected with a right-angle Mixter clamp (Fig. 45–2B). The artery is ligated in continuity with 0-0 silk sutures and divided. For

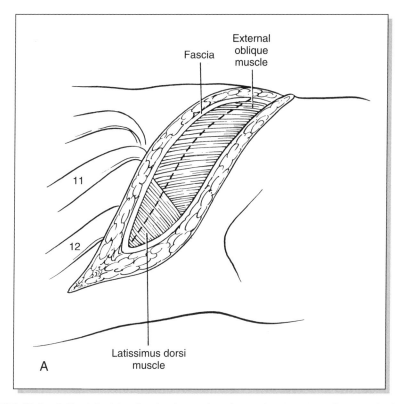

FIGURE 45–2 *A,* Flank incision for simple nephrectomy showing the latissimus dorsi and external oblique muscles to be divided.

Illustration continued on the following page

further security, a 2-0 silk transfixion suture ligature is placed at the proximal end (Fig. 45–2*C*). If any additional arteries are present, these are addressed in a similar fashion.

Next, the renal vein, which lies anterior to the artery, is dissected and doubly ligated in continuity. On the left side, it may be necessary to divide the gonadal, adrenal, and renolumbar veins before addressing the renal vein. The kidney is grasped and delivered into the wound. The ureter is isolated, divided, and ligated with 2-0 silk sutures. The wound is irrigated and hemostasis is achieved. The wound is filled with sterile saline solution and observed for bubbles, which may indicate that the pleural lining has been breached. If bubbles are present, either a chest tube is inserted or a small red Robinson catheter is placed through the pleural defect into the thoracic cavity; the catheter is withdrawn after completion of the wound closure, while the anesthesiologist is expanding the lung. Through a separate stab incision, a 10-mm Jackson-Pratt drain is placed into the cavity.

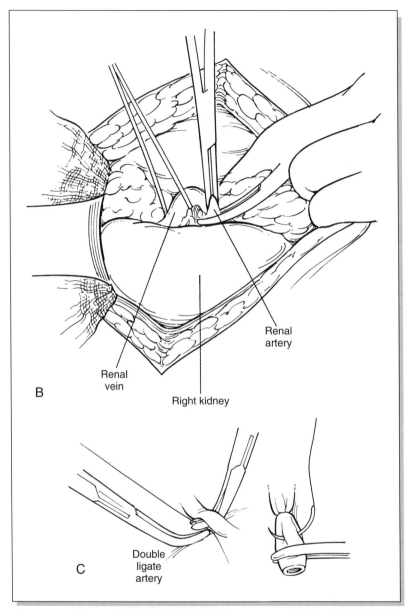

B

Renal
artery

Renal
vein

Right kidney

C

Double
ligate
artery

FIGURE 45–2 *Continued.* *B,* Hilar dissection showing a vessel loop elevating the renal vein to provide access to the renal artery. *C,* Technique of ligating the vessels in continuity and placing a transfixion suture.

CLOSURE   The wound is closed in layers using 2-0 absorbable sutures. The skin is closed with staples.

Radical Nephrectomy

POSITION   The patient is placed in the supine position, and the flank can be slightly elevated by placing a log roll beneath it. The abdomen and the lower chest are prepped and draped in the usual sterile manner. A transabdominal approach is achieved through a subcostal incision based primarily on the side of the nephrectomy, which is adequate for exposure and can be extended across the midline. For a large tumor, particularly at the upper pole, a thoracoabdominal incision may be used. The muscles and fascia of the anterior abdominal wall are incised, and the peritoneal cavity is entered.

EXPOSURE AND OPERATIVE TECHNIQUE   A thorough exploration is performed with particular attention paid to excluding distant metastases and to identifying the presence of coexisting intra-abdominal pathology. A self-retaining retractor system is arranged around the wound, and the anterior abdominal wall is retracted to improve the exposure.

Right-sided Nephrectomy   For right-sided nephrectomy, the peritoneal reflection along the lateral border of the ascending colon and hepatic flexure is sharply divided and retracted medially to display the duodenum. The duodenum is mobilized with the Kocher maneuver to reveal the inferior vena cava. Moist laparotomy pads are placed around the medially rotated colon and duodenum to hold them in position with the retractors. The right renal vein is identified and gently dissected, and a vessel loop is placed around it. Using the vessel loop, the renal vein is carefully lifted up to allow pulsation of the renal artery to be felt beneath it. The main renal and any accessory arteries are carefully isolated and ligated in continuity with 2-0 silk, ensuring that two ligatures are placed proximally. An additional transfixion suture ligature using 3-0 silk should be placed on the proximal stump. The renal vein is not tied until all the renal arteries are dealt with. The renal vein is next ligated in continuity with 0-0 silk ligature and divided. An additional 2-0 silk transfixion suture ligature is placed on the proximal stump. If there are any lumbar veins entering the distal renal vein or the adjacent vena cava, they should also be ligated in continuity.

Once the renal pedicle has been divided, the incision is carried upward and downward anterior to the adventitia in front of the inferior vena cava, with particular care taken to hemoclip small lymph vessels. The fibroadipose and lymphatic tissues are dissected laterally; the tissue over the anterior and lateral surfaces of the inferior vena cava is included with the specimen. The ureter and the right gonadal vein are mobilized sharply to the level of the aortic bifurcation. Each of these structures is individually ligated with 0-0 silk sutures and divided. The gonadal vein is also divided and ligated at the point of its entry into the inferior vena cava.

With the medial aspect of the dissection completed, the peritoneal reflection over the lateral aspect of the kidney is divided and extended from the level of the aortic bifurcation inferiorly to just above the adrenal glands. Gerota's fascia is mobilized off the renal bed, which consists of quadratus lumborum and psoas muscles. A variety of small and large collateral vessels will be encountered and can be either hemoclipped or ligated with 2-0 silk sutures.

After the inferior pole and the lateral aspect of the kidney have been mobilized, the entire specimen is displaced caudally, and large hemoclips are placed to control vessels and lymphatics contained within the adventitial tissue above the adrenal gland. Additional regional lymphadenectomy may be performed, which involves carefully dissecting the lymphatic tissue along the anterior surface of the aorta and vena cava; the lymphadenectomy extends from the level of the adrenal vein to the inferior mesenteric artery.

Left Radical Nephrectomy For left radical nephrectomy, the approach involves division of the peritoneum along the line of Toldt on the lateral aspect of the descending colon. This is carried around the splenic flexure. Beneath it, the splenorenal ligament is divided to mobilize the pancreas and the spleen upward and to the right. These structures can be packed away to the right using moist laparotomy pads. The colon is lifted and reflected medially until the aorta and the anteromedial aspect of the inferior vena cava are clearly visualized. The left renal vein is located and dissected as it arches over the aorta. A vessel loop is placed around the renal vein and lifted upward to provide access to the renal artery, and its branches are ligated in continuity with 2-0 silk and divided. An additional suture ligature using 3-0 silk is placed proximally. A search should be made for accessory renal arteries, which should be dealt in a similar fashion.

Once the renal arteries have been addressed, the renal vein is ligated in continuity with 0-0 silk sutures and divided. Similar to the right-sided nephrectomy, the adventitia and lymphatic tissues are dissected off the anterior wall of the aorta and displaced toward the specimen. The left gonadal vessels and the left ureter are bluntly dissected to the level of the aortic bifurcation and ligated with 2-0 silk and divided. The lateral peritoneal reflection around the border of the kidney is divided, and Gerota's fascia is mobilized off the renal bed. Vessels encountered during the mobilization of the kidney from its bed are hemoclipped and divided. The kidney is retracted inferiorly, and the fibroadipose tissue around the adrenal gland is secured with large hemoclips and divided.

Once the specimen has been removed, a similar limited regional lymphadenectomy along the anterior and lateral surfaces of the aorta can be performed, extending from the superior to the inferior mesenteric artery. The lymphatic tissue lying between the vena cava and the aorta is removed.

If there is preoperative or intraoperative evidence of thrombus within the renal vein, this is dealt with by placing Rummel tourniquets around the inferior vena cava above and below the entry of the renal veins. Alternatively, bleeding from the inferior vena cava can be controlled with vascular clamps. Both renal veins are similarly controlled. The inferior vena cava is lifted, and lumbar veins entering on its deep surface are carefully hemoclipped or tied with 3-0 silk ligatures. After the Rummel tourniquets are tightened, the inferior vena cava is opened longitudinally and the tumor and the cuff of the renal vein from which it is extending are removed. This segment of the inferior vena cava is flushed with heparinized saline, and the venotomy is closed with running 3-0 polypropylene monofilament sutures. The Rummel tourniquets are released, and the venotomy is inspected for leaks.

CLOSURE   The abdominal musculature is closed in layers with continuous 2-0 absorbable sutures. Skin is approximated with staples.

CHAPTER 46

Orchiectomy

EMBRYOLOGY   In the fourth week of gestation, the genital or gonadal ridges appear on each side of the midline between the mesonephros and the dorsal mesentery. These ridges are formed by proliferation of the coelomic epithelium and condensation of the underlying mesenchyme. The coelomic epithelium proliferates and penetrates the underlying mesenchyme to form numerous irregularly shaped cords, called the primitive sex cords. The sex cords eventually lose connection from the overlying coelomic epithelium by the development of a thick fibrous connective tissue, called the tunica albuginea. The primitive sex cells, called the primordial germ cells, are initially located in the mesoderm surrounding the allantoic diverticulum. By the third week of gestation these germ cells migrate by ameboid movement through the dorsal mesentery of the hindgut to reach the gonadal ridge by the fifth week. The primitive sex cords surround the invading primordial germ cells and form anastomosing branches at the hilum, called the rete testis. The rete testis in turn communicates with 5 to 15 efferent ductules that continue as the convoluted epididymis and then the ductus deferens. The efferent ductules, epididymis, and vas deferens are all derivatives of the wolffian duct (mesonephric duct).

Attached to the caudal part of the testis is the ligamentous remnant of the mesonephros, known as gubernaculum testis. During the second month of development body growth occurs rapidly, and because the gubernaculum fails to elongate concomitantly, the testis descends caudally. By the seventh week the testis comes to lie adjacent to the inguinal canal, and before birth it has descended into the scrotum.

ANATOMY The two testes are oval organs lying suspended within the scrotum by the spermatic cord. Each testis is surrounded by a tough fibrous capsule, called the tunica albuginea. Attached to the posterolateral surface of the testes is the epididymis, whereas the vas deferens lies on the medial aspect. Each testis is covered with the tunica vaginalis, which is a continuation of the processus vaginalis, the internal spermatic fascia, the cremasteric fascia, and the external spermatic fascia. All these layers are in essence a continuation of the coverings around the spermatic cord. The superficial fascia of the abdominal wall is replaced within the scrotal wall by smooth muscle called dartos muscle. Scarpa's fascia of the anterior abdominal wall continues within the scrotum as Colles' fascia. Colles' fascia also forms a median scrotal septum that forms a partition between the two testes.

The blood supply of the testes is via the testicular artery, which is a branch of the aorta. The venous blood drains through the pampiniform plexus that forms the testicular veins. The right testicular vein drains into the inferior vena cava and the left into the left renal vein. The lymphatic drainage of the wall of the scrotum and the layers surrounding the testes is into superficial nodes; the lymphatic drainage of the testes passes with the arteries to the para-aortic nodes.

The spermatic cord has three coverings and contains three nerves, three arteries, and three other structures. The three layers are the internal spermatic fascia, which is a continuation of the transversalis fascia; the cremasteric fascia and muscle, arising from the internal oblique; and the external spermatic fascia, arising from the external oblique. The nerves are the ilioinguinal, the genital branch of the genitofemoral, and the sympathetic nerves. The three arteries are the testicular arteries, arising from the aorta; the cremasteric artery, which is a branch of the inferior epigastric artery; and the artery to the vas deferens, a branch of the inferior vesical artery. The other three structures are the lymphatic vessels, the pampiniform plexus of veins, and the vas deferens.

SPECIAL PREOPERATIVE PREPARATION The approach for orchiectomy depends on whether the procedure is being performed for benign or malignant conditions. Simple bilateral orchiectomy is often undertaken for metastatic carcinoma of the prostate. For malignant primary tumors of the testis, radical orchiectomy is performed.

Operative Procedure

Simple Orchiectomy

POSITION The patient is placed in the supine position, and the genitalia are prepped and draped in sterile fashion

INCISION   Bilateral orchidectomy can be performed using either a single midline incision or a transverse incision extending across the midline.

EXPOSURE AND OPERATIVE TECHNIQUE   The scrotal skin is incised with a scalpel. After this, the dartos muscle and the subsequent underlying tissues are divided by electrocautery. Once the tunica vaginalis is incised, the testis is withdrawn from its sac and through the incision. The cord is clamped and divided. Proximally the cord is doubly ligated with 0 silk sutures. An additional 2-0 silk transfixion suture ligature is also applied. A similar procedure is performed for the other testis. The soft tissue is approximated in layers with interrupted or continuous 3-0 absorbable sutures. The scrotal skin is closed with a subcuticular 3-0 absorbable suture. Alternatively, the scrotum can be closed with full-thickness interrupted 3-0 absorbable sutures.

Radical Orchiectomy

POSITION   The patient is placed in the supine position, and the genitalia and the inguinal region are prepped and draped in a sterile fashion.

INCISION   An inguinal skin incision is made that is the same as for inguinal herniorrhaphy (see Chapter 13).

EXPOSURE AND OPERATIVE TECHNIQUE   The incision is carried on through the subcutaneous tissue until the external oblique fascia is identified. This is incised and opened toward the external ring. The spermatic cord is freed and clamped at the level of the internal ring using a rubber-shod clamp or by tightening the looped one-half-inch Penrose drain (Fig. 46–1). The testis is pulled up from the scrotum. If the testis clearly feels and appears grossly abnormal, radical orchiectomy should be done. If there is doubt, the tunica vaginalis is opened and an incisional biopsy of the testis is undertaken. If a tumor is confirmed either by frozen section or by gross appearance, the cord is doubly clamped at the level of the internal ring. A separate clamp is placed distally and the cord is divided. The cord is ligated with 0-0 silk sutures. An additional 2-0 silk transfixion suture ligature is placed to transfix the cord. The wound is irrigated with sterile saline.

CLOSURE   The external aponeurosis is closed with 2-0 absorbable sutures. Scarpa's fascia is approximated with 3-0 absorbable sutures, and the skin is closed with subcuticular 4-0 absorbable sutures and reinforced with Steri-Strips.

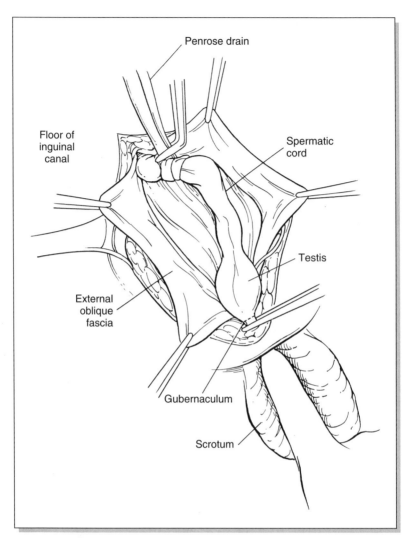

Penrose drain

Floor of
inguinal
canal

Spermatic
cord

Testis

External
oblique
fascia

Gubernaculum

Scrotum

FIGURE 46–1 The spermatic cord is clamped at the level of the internal ring and then the testis delivered from the scrotum into the wound.

CHAPTER 47

Orchidopexy

EMBRYOLOGY AND ANATOMY   See Chapter 46.

SPECIAL PREOPERATIVE PREPARATION   Except for an adequate history and physical, no special preoperative preparation is necessary.

Operative Procedure

POSITION   The patient is placed in the supine position and undergoes general anesthesia with endotracheal intubation. The lower abdomen, genitalia, and upper thigh are prepped with antiseptic solution and draped in a sterile fashion. The surgeon evaluates the true status of the undescended testis while the child is under anesthesia, in particular assessing the position and the mobility of the testis.

INCISION   A skin-crease incision is made directly over the inguinal canal, which has its center point approximately 2 cm above the femoral pulse (Fig. 47–1).

EXPOSURE AND OPERATIVE TECHNIQUE   The skin, subcutaneous tissue, and superficial fascia are carefully incised. If the testis is ectopic within the superficial inguinal pouch, it can now be easily identified. The testis is lifted and freed on the lateral aspect to identify the cord that is seen passing through the superficial inguinal ring. However, if the testis is within the inguinal canal, it will not be seen until the external oblique fascia is incised.

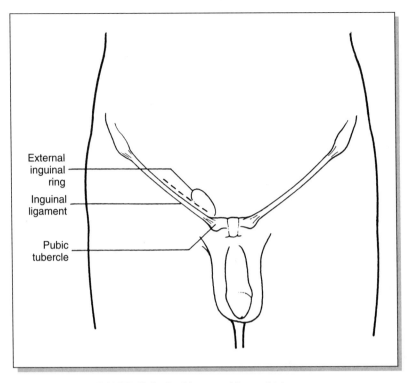

FIGURE 47-1 Incision used for orchidopexy.

The superficial inguinal ring is first identified and the external oblique aponeurosis incised with a no. 15 scalpel. The edges of this small stab incision are carefully grasped with fine hemostats. Under direct vision, the external oblique fascia is opened from the superficial inguinal ring to the lateral aspect of the incision. Particular care is taken in identifying the ilioinguinal nerve, which should be preserved. A blunt-tipped self-retaining retractor is inserted to hold apart the edges of the external oblique aponeurosis. In most patients, the testis should now be obvious or should already have been identified if present within the superficial inguinal pouch.

At the distal end of the testis, a mixture of fibroadipose tissue is carefully dissected, leaving the gubernaculum, which is a tough strand that must be clamped, divided, and ligated with 3-0 absorbable sutures. The ligature on the testicular side can be left long for subsequent traction. Using this ligature, the testis is held up and the strands of cremasteric muscles are sharply divided with electrocautery (Fig. 47–2). As the cremasteric fibers are divided, the margins of the internal ring will become clear. Next, the anterolateral aspect of the cord is inspected for the thin-walled

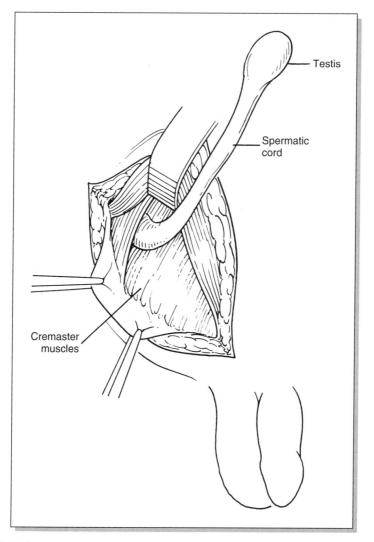

FIGURE 47–2 Mobilized testis and the spermatic cord seen within the inguinal canal.

hernia sac. The sac is carefully dissected from the cord structures with a fine Halsted mosquito hemostat. The sac is freed to the level of the internal ring, whereupon it is twisted and transfixed at the neck with 3-0 absorbable sutures. The excess sac is excised. If at this stage the testes can reach the scrotum, further mobilization is not required. However, if further length is required, small retractors are inserted in the lateral aspect of the deep ring. Using a Kittner dissector, a plane is developed between the peritoneum and the testicular vessels. Usually there are several fibrous strands on the lateral aspect of the vessels. As these strands are divided, the cord will elongate further. If further mobilization is necessary, the internal ring can be opened on its medial border up to the level of inferior epigastric vessels. If at this stage the length of the cord still appears short, a staged procedure may need to be considered.

Once adequate length of the cord has been established, the testis must be fixed in the scrotum using the dartos pouch method. The index finger is passed down into the scrotum from the groin wound (Fig. 47–3A). A small transverse incision is made at the lowest part of the scrotum. A subdartos pouch is created between the skin and the loose fascia within the scrotum. With a fine Halsted mosquito hemostat a defect is made within the loose fascia, and the previously tagged suture at the distal end of the testis is grasped. The testis and the cord are brought through the fascial defect, with care taken to ensure that the vessels and vas are not twisted during this maneuver. The testis is gently manipulated into the pouch. The scrotal incision is closed with interrupted 3-0 absorbable suture (Fig. 47–3B). With one of these sutures, a superficial bite of the testis is taken. If the internal ring has been widened, it is snugly closed with interrupted 3-0 absorbable suture.

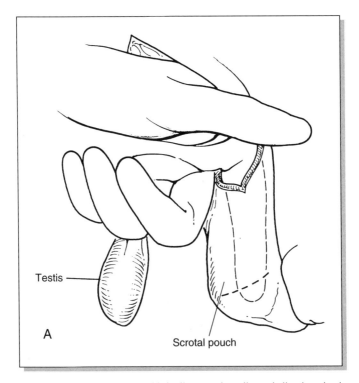

Testis

A

Scrotal pouch

FIGURE 47–3 A, A finger is passed into the scrotum though the inguinal wound

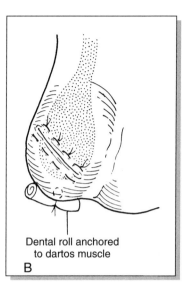

FIGURE 47–3 *Continued.* *B,* The testis is anchored in a subdartos pouch.

Dental roll anchored
to dartos muscle
B

CLOSURE   The external oblique is closed with continuous 3-0 absorbable sutures. The superficial fascia (Scarpa's fascia), which is quite prominent in young adults and children, is also approximated with 3-0 absorbable sutures. The skin is approximated with subcuticular 4-0 absorbable sutures. The skin closure is reinforced with Steri-Strips.

CHAPTER 48

Radical Cystectomy

EMBRYOLOGY   As described in Chapter 36, the cloaca is divided by a ridge of mesodermal tissue, known as urorectal septum, into a posterior anorectal canal and an anterior primitive urogenital sinus. The primitive urogenital sinus can be divided into three parts: upper vesical, middle pelvic, and distal phallic. The dilated upper part of the primitive urogenital sinus forms the transitional epithelium of the bladder, whereas the adjacent mesenchyme forms the muscular wall. The vesical segment is continuous with the allantois, which eventually obliterates to form the urachus, which connects the apex of the bladder to the umbilicus. In adults the urachus is represented by the median umbilical ligament. The trigone of the bladder is derived from mesonephric tissue, though its lining originates from the endoderm of the urogenital sinus. The narrow pelvic part of the urogenital sinus forms the membranous and prostatic urethra. The phallic part of the urogenital sinus gives rise to the penile urethra in males and a small segment of the urethra and the vestibule in females.

ANATOMY   The bladder is a muscular reservoir for urine that lies within the pelvic cavity as an extraperitoneal organ. When the bladder is empty, it is pyramidal with an apex, a base, a superior surface, and two anterolateral surfaces. The apex lies directly behind the symphysis pubis. From it emerges the remnant of the urachus, known as the median umbilical ligament. The base of the bladder is triangular, with the ureters entering the bladder at the two lateral angles. The urethra emerges from the inferior angle of the base, which is also the neck of the bladder.

The internal surface of the base of the bladder is referred to as the trigone; the mucosa at the trigone is smooth and firmly adheres to the underlying muscular layer. The peritoneum covers the superior surface of the bladder and partly covers the upper part of the posterior surface. Lying against the lower part of the posterior surface are the ampule of the vas deferens and the seminal vesicles. The bladder is surrounded by pelvic fascia, which is condensed around the neck to form the pubovesical and puboprostatic ligaments anteriorly, the lateral ligaments extending to the lateral pelvic wall, and the posterior ligament extending toward the rectum.

The arterial supply of the bladder originates from the superior and inferior vesical branches of the internal iliac artery. The venous drainage flows into the internal iliac vein via the vesical plexus. The lymphatic drainage from the bladder is into the internal and external iliac lymph nodes. The bladder is innervated through the lumbar nerve segments. The sympathetic fibers arise from the first and second lumbar segments, whereas the parasympathetic fibers arise from sacral segments two, three, and four.

SPECIAL PREOPERATIVE EVALUATION A thorough pulmonary and cardiac evaluation must be undertaken. The patient is instructed on breathing exercises and, importantly, is seen by the stoma therapist to be familiarized with urinary diversion and the associated appliances. The enterostomal therapists also mark the sites for the stoma. Mechanical bowel preparation using either Nichol's prep or polyethylene glycol-electrolyte solution (GoLYTELY) is provided.

Operative Procedure

POSITION The patient is placed in modified Lloyd-Davies position, with the legs abducted and slightly flexed at the hip and the knee joint. The patient undergoes general anesthesia with endotracheal intubation. An epidural catheter may be inserted for postoperative pain management. A Foley catheter is placed within the bladder. Pneumatic compression devices are applied to both lower extremities. A nasogastric tube is also inserted.

INCISION A lower midline incision extending from the symphysis pubis to above the umbilicus is made and may be extended to the xiphoid as needed. The linea alba is incised, and the rectus muscle is retracted laterally.

EXPOSURE AND OPERATIVE TECHNIQUE In the upper part of the incision, the posterior rectus sheath and the peritoneum are divided. As this incision is continued inferiorly, the urachal remnant is identified and divided.

A Kocher clamp is placed on the transected segment for traction. A thorough intra-abdominal exploration is undertaken to evaluate the extent of the malignant process. The liver is also assessed for the presence of metastatic disease. Next, a self-retaining retractor system is placed and the abdominal wall is retracted laterally. The patient is placed in a slight Trendelenburg position, and the small bowel is carefully packed toward the upper abdomen, covered with moist laparotomy pads, and held in place with a large retractor.

Dissection begins by dividing the peritoneal lining along the lateral edges of the bladder. Next, the sigmoid and descending colon are mobilized by incising the avascular line of Toldt along the left paracolic gutter. This incision in the left gutter extends from the sacral promontory to the level of the lower pole of the left kidney. The peritoneal lining on the medial surface of the sigmoid colon is incised and extended toward the right side of the pelvic inlet. After incision of the peritoneal reflection, both ureters are identified and mobilized at the level of the common iliac artery. Two large hemoclips are placed across both ureters, which are then divided. A 3-0 silk stay suture is placed at the edge of the proximal end of the ureters for traction. The left ureter, which is to be used for urinary diversion, is brought under the sigmoid mesocolon to lie alongside the right ureter. During ureteral mobilization meticulous preservation of their blood supply is achieved by avoiding skeletonization.

Pelvic lymphadenectomy is commenced by exposing the aortic bifurcation and skeletonizing the external iliac artery and vein. The limits of the lymphadenectomy are as follows: laterally the genitofemoral nerve, medially the pectineal ligament, and distally the deep circumflex iliac vein. All the fibroadipose and lymphatic tissues within the boundaries described above are dissected and swept toward the bladder to be removed as an en bloc resection. After skeletonization of the external iliac vessels and the obturator fossa, mobilization of the bladder is started by undertaking the lateral dissection. The internal iliac artery is dissected, and the first branch, the superior gluteal artery, is identified and preserved. Distal to this level, the internal iliac artery is carefully dissected, and using a Mixter right-angle clamp 0-0 silk ligatures are passed. The internal iliac artery is ligated and divided, and an additional 2-0 silk transfixion suture ligature is placed on the proximal transected end of the vessel. In this fashion, both the lateral pedicles are divided (Fig. 48–1A). Alternatively, the lateral pedicles can be conveniently divided using an endovascular stapler.

Having addressed the lateral pedicles, attention is now turned to posterior dissection. The bladder is retracted anteriorly with a deep St. Mark's retractor to visualize the rectovesical pouch of Douglas. The previously incised peritoneum along the sigmoid colon is extended along the lateral aspect of the rectum and carried anteriorly into the pouch of Douglas. The incision in the cul-de-sac should be closer to the anterior rectal wall rather

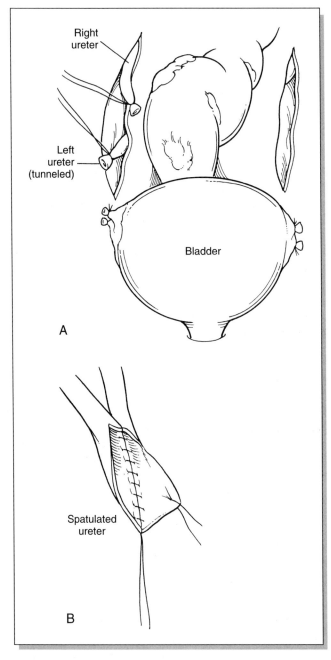

FIGURE 48–1 *A,* The lateral pedicle of the bladder has been divided and ligated. The left ureter has been tunneled under the sigmoid mesocolon to lie adjacent to the right ureter. *B,* The ends of the ureters are spatulated and then sutured together.

than to the bladder to ensure entering into Denonvilliers' space. This allows the rectum to be easily dissected away from the bladder, seminal vesicles, and prostate gland in men and from the posterior vaginal wall in women. In so doing, the posterior pedicle extending from the bladder to the lateral side of the rectum on each side is delineated. The pedicles are hemoclipped and divided all the way to the endopelvic fascia in men. The endopelvic fascia is incised circumferentially around the prostate.

Anterior dissection involves mobilizing the prostate from the pubis. The puboprostatic ligaments are isolated, hemoclipped, and divided close to the pubis. With a Mixter right-angle clamp, the dorsal vein of the penis is carefully freed, ligated in continuity using 2-0 silk, and divided. Dissection is continued beyond the prostate, and an umbilical tape is passed around the urethra. The urethra is clamped and divided near the prostate. The rectourethralis muscle is sharply divided with electrocautery. Because the specimen has been circumferentially dissected, it should now be free except for any remaining connections to the endopelvic fascia.

The proximal ends of both ureters are carefully mobilized for 3 to 4 cm with their vascular sheath preserved (Fig. 48–1B). It is vital that the adventitia of the ureter containing its delicate blood supply not be excised to the bare ureter. The left ureter is passed beneath the sigmoid mesocolon, with care taken that it is not twisted or angulated.

With both ureters now ready for anastomosis to the intestine, attention is directed to fashioning the ileal segment. Before proceeding with isolation of the ileal segment, an appendectomy is performed. Approximately 6 to 8 inches (~20 cm) from the ileocecal valve, an 8- to 10-inch (20- to 25-cm) segment of ileum is selected. In obese patients, a slightly longer segment is required. The distal and proximal ends of segment are divided with a GIA-55 stapler. Adjacent to this division, the mesentery and its vessels are divided and ligated for a depth of approximately 2 or 3 cm. For purpose of subsequent identification, the proximal end of the isolated ileal segment is marked with a 3-0 silk stay suture. Continuity of the bowel is restored with an end-to-end anastomosis in two layers, which is performed anterior to the vascular pedicle of the isolated ileal segment.

Attention is now turned to creating the anastomosis of the ureters at the proximal end of the ileal segment. The left ureter is brought in proximity to the ileal segment, and the anastomosis is begun by placing 3-0 silk sutures between the ureteric adventitia and the serosa of the ileal segment. A small 4- to 5-mm enterotomy is made within the bowel, and a mucosa-to-mucosa full-thickness anastomosis using 4-0 absorbable sutures is performed. Before the ureteroileal anastomosis is completed, a small ureteric stent is passed into each ureter and brought out through the distal end of the ileal segment. After the inner layer of 4-0 absorbable sutures has been placed, three or four fine 4-0 silk sutures are added to complete the outer row, which incorporates the serosa and the periureteric tissue containing the blood supply of the ureter. During the anastomosis there must be minimal manipulation of the distal end of the ureter with instruments. The right ureter is anastomosed in a similar fashion approximately 1 cm away from the left ureteroileal anastomosis.

After the ureteroileal anastomosis is completed, the distal end of the ileal segment is ready to be delivered through the external stoma (Fig. 48–2). At the preoperatively determined stoma site, a circular skin incision is made and a segment of subcutaneous adipose tissue is excised. An incision is made through the fascial and muscular layers down to and through the peritoneum. The size of the opening through layers of the abdominal wall should allow two fingers to pass through comfortably. After the opening has been completed, a long Babcock clamp is inserted through it from outside, and the end of the ileal segment is gently grasped and drawn through the opening, with care taken that there is no twisting of the mesentery. A standard Brook's ileostomy is created. At completion, the segment is inspected, particularly to ensure that there is no tension.

The defect within the mesentery formed by the end-to-end ileal anastomosis over the vascular pedicle of the ileal segment is approximated with continuous 3-0 absorbable sutures. It is best to postpone this part of the procedure until the external stoma has been constructed.

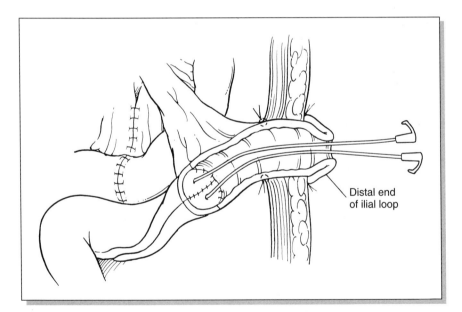

Distal end
of ilial loop

FIGURE 48–2 The common ureteric orifice is anastomosed to the ileal loop with stents in place. The ileal loop is brought through the anterior abdominal wall as Brook's ileostomy.

The abdomen is now irrigated with sterile saline. Hemostasis is achieved.

CLOSURE   The abdomen is closed by approximating the linea alba with continuous 1-0 monofilament nonabsorbable sutures. The skin is approximated with staples. A transparent stoma bag is placed over the ileostomy and connected to a bag for accurate measurement of urinary output.

CHAPTER 49

Circumcision

PREOPERATIVE PREPARATION No preoperative preparation is needed, except for ensuring that the patient can undergo general anesthesia.

ANESTHESIA General anesthetic is administered.

Operative Procedure

EXPOSURE AND OPERATIVE TECHNIQUE For children who may have phimosis with a prior history of recurrent balanitis, the opening in the foreskin must be gently opened with a fine Halsted mosquito hemostat. The foreskin is retracted backward to the limb of the coronal sulcus. Any further adhesions between the inner mucosal layer and the glans are bluntly separated with moist gauze. In children, the coronal sulcus is marked on the foreskin with indelible pen. The foreskin is stretched and, to facilitate hemostasis, is gently compressed with a straight clamp at the marking. At this level the foreskin is sharply divided with straight scissors. Alternatively, two Halsted mosquito hemostats are placed at the 2 o'clock and 10 o'clock positions. With fine curved scissors, a dorsal slit is made down to the level of the coronal sulcus (Fig. 49–1*A*). Next a ventral slit is made to the level of the frenulum. The foreskin that is now in two halves can be excised with Metzenbaum scissors at the level of the coronal sulcus. The frenular vessel is picked up with fine Halsted mosquito forceps and ligated with 3-0 absorbable sutures (Fig. 49–1*B*). Any other bleeding points are also ligated with 3-0 absorbable sutures. Use of electrocautery must be avoided because it runs the risk of deep coagulation of vessels in the base of the penis.

Occasionally, an excess of inner mucosal layer remains. This can be trimmed with fine Metzenbaum scissors to leave a 2- to 4-mm rim of tissue around the coronal sulcus. The skin is aligned to this mucosa, ensuring that no twisting has occurred. These two layers are sutured together with interrupted 3-0 absorbable sutures such as plain catgut (Fig. 49–1*C*). Any persistent bleeding can be addressed by placing interrupted simple sutures between the mucosa and the skin. A nonadherent dressing is placed around the wound.

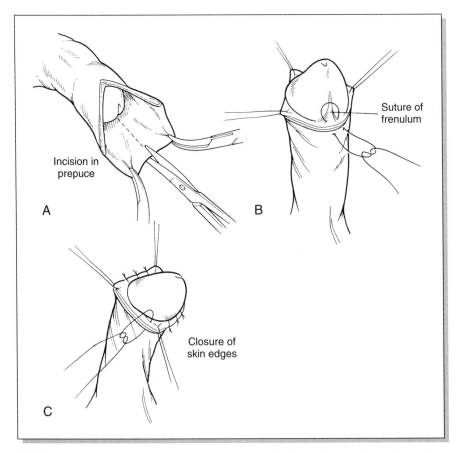

FIGURE 49–1 *A,* With a fine-curved scissors, a dorsal slit is made down to the level of the coronal sulcus. *B,* The frenular vessel is ligated with 3-0 absorbable suture. *C,* The skin is aligned to the mucosa, and these two layers are sutured together with interrupted 3-0 absorbable suture such as plain catgut.

Gynecology

CHAPTER 50

Total Abdominal Hysterectomy

EMBRYOLOGY The müllerian or paramesonephric duct arises as a longitudinal invagination of the coelomic epithelium on the anterolateral surface of the urogenital ridge. Caudally, the two müllerian ducts grow in the medial direction and fuse together in the midline to form the uterine canal, which continues to grow in a caudal direction. At the point where it comes in contact with the posterior wall of the urogenital sinus (pelvic part), it causes a small swelling, called the müllerian tubercle. The fused common duct gives rise to the body and cervix of the uterus. The horizontal part of the müllerian duct just proximal to the fusion develops into the uterine tubes.

Shortly after formation, the müllerian tubercle begins to proliferate to form the sinovaginal bulb (vaginal plate). This solid plate encircles the caudal end of the fused müllerian ducts and increases in length. The vaginal plate develops a lumen at its caudal end, and by the fifth month of development the entire plate has canalized. The part surrounding the caudal end of the uterus (i.e., cervix) forms the vaginal fornices. The lumen of the vagina remains separated from that of the urogenital sinus by a thin tissue plate, known as the hymen.

ANATOMY The uterus is a pear-shaped organ lying within the pelvic cavity between the rectum posteriorly and the bladder anteriorly. In its usual anteverted position, the uterus is directed forward with its long axis at 90 degrees to the vagina. The uterus is divided into a fundus, body, and cervix. The segment of the uterus that lies above the entry of the fallopian tube is known as the fundus. The body is the main part of the uterus and has a cavity, which is triangular in the coronal section. The body of the uterus is continuous inferiorly with the cervix. The convex cervical canal communicates superiorly with the cavity of the uterine body with the vagina through the external os. The entire uterus is covered with peritoneal lining except anteriorly, where at the level of the internal os the peritoneum passes forward onto the superior surface of the bladder. The peritoneum drapes laterally over the fallopian tubes and passes laterally to the lateral pelvic wall to form the broad ligaments of the uterus. The uterus is supported primarily by the levator ani muscles and by three paired ligaments: the uterosacral, the lateral cervical (cardinal), and the pubocervical ligaments. The round ligament of the uterus is a remnant of the gubernaculum and extends from the superolateral angle of the uterus through the broad ligament and the internal ring to end in the labium majus.

The uterus receives its blood supply from the uterine artery, a branch of the internal iliac artery that runs medially in the base of the broad ligament and crosses above the ureter at the level of the internal os. The artery then extends, within the broad ligament, along the lateral border of the uterus to anastomose with the ovarian artery. Venous drainage is via the uterine and internal iliac veins. Lymphatic drainage is primarily to the external and common iliac nodes. However, some lymphatics vessels also drain along the round ligament to the superficial inguinal nodes, and others drain with the ovarian vessels into the para-aortic nodes. The nerve supply of the uterus is derived from branches of the pelvic plexus.

PREOPERATIVE PREPARATION   The cardiovascular and respiratory systems must be adequately evaluated. Perioperative antibiotics are administered. General anesthesia is provided with endotracheal intubation. A nasogastric tube and Foley catheter are inserted. If preoperative work-up reveals an extensive pelvic inflammatory process that may make identification of the ureters difficult, perioperative placement of ureteral stents should be considered. Because the vagina will be entered during the procedure, it is cleansed with dilute Betadine solution. Perioperative administration of 5000 units of heparin subcutaneously and the use of sequential pneumatic compression devices are recommended for prevention of deep vein thrombosis.

Operative Procedure

POSITION   The patient is usually placed in the supine position, and because access to the vagina from below may be required, the legs are placed on stirrups.

INCISION   A low midline incision extending from the pubis to just above the umbilicus is made, and the abdominal cavity is entered.

EXPOSURE AND OPERATIVE TECHNIQUE   After a systematic exploration of the abdominal cavity, the patient is placed in the Trendelenburg position. A self-retaining retractor system is placed for exposure. The small bowel is packed superiorly to provide adequate exposure of the pelvic structures. Straight Kocher clamps are placed across the cornual portion of the uterus such that they occlude the round ligament, fallopian tube, and uterine and ovarian vessels. Using these clamps the uterus is retracted upward, thus placing the structures within the broad ligament under tension. The round ligament is divided, and the proximal end is ligated with 0-0 silk sutures. These sutures are tagged with a hemostat to provide lateral traction (Fig. 50–1A).

Once the round ligament has been divided, the peritoneum over the anterolateral aspect of the broad ligament is incised along the uterus and parallel to the fallopian tubes to expose the underlying avascular area. At

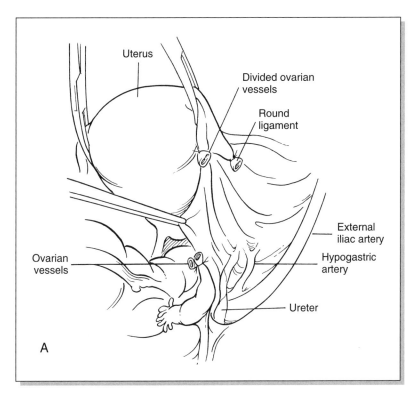

FIGURE 50–1   A, The round ligament and the fallopian tubes have been divided. Clamps are placed at the cornu of the uterus for traction. The relationship of the ureter to the uterine artery arising from the hypogastric artery can be seen.

Illustration continued on the following page

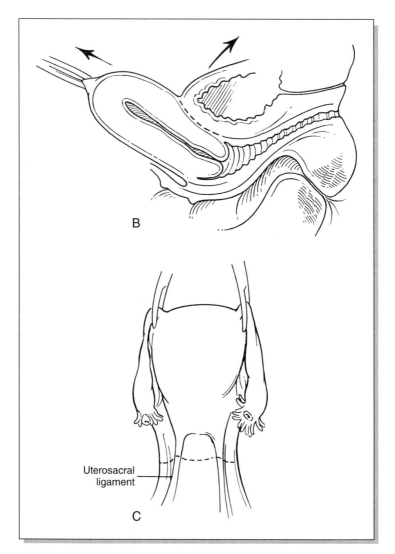

FIGURE 50–1 *Continued.* *B.* The plane of dissection between the uterus and the bladder is shown in sagittal section. *C,* Posterior view of the uterus demonstrating the uterosacral ligament.

this stage the ovarian vessels are carefully dissected with a Mixter right-angle clamp, ligated with 0-0 silk sutures, and divided. Alternatively, the vascular pedicle can be secured with an endovascular linear stapler. If the ovaries are to be preserved, the fallopian tubes are divided and ligated, leaving the ovarian vessels intact (see Fig. 50–1*A*). Next, the ureter is exposed on both sides, from the pelvic brim down to the level of the uterine artery within the pelvis.

Attention is now directed to mobilizing the bladder away from the anterior surface of the uterus, cervix, and upper vagina (Fig. 50–1*B*). This dissection is initiated by first dividing the vesicouterine peritoneum that joins the lateral openings previously made in the peritoneum of the broad ligaments. With the use of sharp electrocautery dissection, the areolar tissue between the endopelvic fascia and the bladder is divided. During the anterior dissection the cervix is intermittently palpated to gauge the length of the distal dissection. At the level of the cervix, on the lateral aspect, the uterine artery can be seen traveling medially to the cervix. Here the previously exposed ureters can be seen passing beneath the uterine artery.

When the anterior dissection has been completed, the uterus is retracted upward and anteriorly. Next the posterior peritoneal covering of the broad ligament is incised on both sides and extended into peritoneum of the rectovaginal cul-de-sac. With electrocautery the strong uterosacral ligaments are divided (Fig. 50–1*C*); this allows clear visualization of the cardinal ligaments containing the transverse portion of the uterine artery. While keeping the ureters under view, the cardinal ligaments are clamped on both sides and divided. The proximal part of the cardinal ligament is suture ligated with 2-0 silk sutures. Blind clamping in this region is a frequent cause for iatrogenic injury to the ureters. With the cardinal and the uterosacral ligaments divided on each side, the uterus is retracted upward and anteriorly while simultaneously posterior and downward traction is applied on the rectum. This maneuver facilitates identification of the plane between the uterus and the rectum, and the plane is carefully developed to the level of the posterior vaginal fornices.

When the circumferential dissection of the uterus at the level of the cervix has been completed, this area is carefully examined to ensure that the upper part of the vagina has been carefully cleared from the bladder, rectum, and ureters. The uterus can now be removed by dividing the vaginal wall close to the cervix. The resulting vaginal cuff is grasped with Allis clamps and closed with a continuous 2-0 absorbable suture. To ensure support for the vagina after hysterectomy, approximating the pubocervical fascia to the endopelvic fascia anteriorly and the uterosacral ligaments posteriorly restores the upper pelvic diaphragm. Laterally the cardinal ligament is also included. The pelvis is examined to ensure that the ureters, bladder, and rectum have not been injured during the dissection. The pelvis is then re-peritonealized with continuous 3-0 absorbable sutures without leaving any defects that could cause postoperative small bowel obstruction. If complete closure is not feasible, it is wise to avoid re-peritonealizing the pelvis. If the peritoneum is to be reapproximated, the ureters must be identified during each passage of the needle through the two leaves of peritoneum.

CLOSURE The linea alba is closed with continuous 1-0 monofilament nonabsorbable sutures. The skin is approximated with staples.

Index